ARE YOU WATCHING YOUR FAT INTAKE?
TRYING TO MAINTAIN A HEALTHY LIFESTYLE?

COOK WITH CONFIDENCE WITH
CORINNE T. NETZER'S
**COMPLETE BOOK OF FOOD COUNTS
COOKBOOK SERIES**
DON'T MISS . . .

RICE NOODLES WITH FRESH GINGERED TUNA
An Asian-oriented salad that is both low in fat and
undeniably delicious. 315 calories; 23.0 grams protein; 51.0 grams carbohydrates; 1.8 grams fat; 46.5
milligrams cholesterol; 145 milligrams sodium

SPICY EGGPLANT AND ANGEL HAIR PASTA
The secret of this low fat but flavorful dish is to use
either small lavender Asian eggplants or tiny deep
purple Italian eggplants. They are delicate in flavor—
not bitter—and the red pepper flakes give this dish
its kick! 260 calories; 8.0 grams protein; 48.5 grams
carbohydrates; 3.5 grams fat; 1.0 milligrams cholesterol; 35 milligrams sodium

CHICKEN AND RICOTTA PIZZA WITH TOMATOES
AND BELL PEPPER
Who would think we could afford to eat a rich and
satisfying pizza while watching our arteries, not to
mention our waistlines? We can with this one. 260
calories; 13.0 grams protein; 35.0 grams carbohydrates; 7.8 grams fat; 20.5 milligrams cholesterol;
185 milligrams sodium

100 LOW FAT PASTA AND GRAIN RECIPES

THE COMPLETE BOOK OF
FOOD COUNTS COOKBOOK SERIES

100 LOW FAT PASTA AND GRAIN RECIPES

Corinne T. Netzer

A Dell Book

Published by
Dell Publishing
a division of
Bantam Doubleday Dell Publishing Group, Inc.
1540 Broadway
New York, New York 10036

ISBN: 0-440-22337-7

Printed in the United States of America

Published simultaneously in Canada

April 1997

10 9 8 7 6 5 4 3 2 1

OPM

CONTENTS

INTRODUCTION

Delicious! Delicious! Delicious! This is one of six books that comprise my Complete Book of Food Counts Cookbook Series—which also includes *100 Low Fat Chicken and Turkey Recipes, 100 Low Fat Fish and Shellfish Recipes, 100 Low Fat Vegetable and Legume Recipes, 100 Low Fat Soup and Stew Recipes,* and *100 Low Fat Small Meal and Salad Recipes.* And all the recipes are *delicious*!

We are all aware of the need to reduce the fat in our diets, and ordinarily this would mean a sacrifice in taste. How many of us have had the misfortune to sample some very forgettable low fat dishes, where the overriding concern was only the fat content? It is my belief that no matter how ''good'' something is for you, you will not continue to eat it if it doesn't *taste* good, and this will almost certainly defeat your diet.

Every recipe in this book has been tested and sampled so that each dish is as good tasting as it is good for you. Low fat ingredients were not used automatically because they might fit or seemed right. Everything was tried out, because not all ingredients are interchangeable—and what might make sense in theory or at the drawing board may not please the palate.

Here you will find wonderful dishes—both plain and fancy—simple fare to eat and serve on a daily basis, and simply elegant fare that you will be proud to serve on any special occasion. Attention has been paid to the use of herbs and spices, but all the ingredients in these recipes can be found either in your cupboard or in the supermarket.

Good eating!

CTN

SOUPS AND CHOWDERS

LOW FAT CHICKEN STOCK

This stock serves as the base for any number of dishes, as you'll see as you look through this book, and alone it's a wonderful and welcome consomme. For a delicious chicken noodle soup, just add two or three ounces of thin noodles and a bit of cooked diced chicken—let it simmer until the soup is reduced slightly and the noodles are tender. For chicken rice soup, substitute rice for the noodles; for chicken vegetable soup, add onions, carrots, celery, peas, etc.

For future-use convenience, freeze the stock in ice cube trays (remove when frozen and place in plastic bag) or in one-cup portions to use in recipes; it will keep for about a month. Or refrigerate the stock for up to one week.

  2 pounds chicken parts (backs, wings, necks)
 10 cups water
 $^1/_2$ cup dry white wine, optional
  1 large onion, quartered
  2 large carrots, coarsely chopped
  2 large stalks celery, with tops, coarsely chopped
  1 bay leaf
 $^1/_2$ teaspoon whole peppercorns
  8 sprigs fresh parsley
    Salt to taste

1. Combine all ingredients in a soup pot and bring to a boil. Cover, reduce heat to very low and simmer

for about 3 hours, skimming stock as necessary. Remove from heat and let cool to room temperature.

2. Strain stock and discard solids or reserve for other use.

3. Cover and refrigerate stock for at least 4 hours or until very well chilled.

4. Skim off hardened surface fat and discard. Stock is ready to be used or may be refrigerated or frozen in airtight containers for later use.

MAKES ABOUT 8 CUPS

Per 1 cup serving: 25 calories; 1.0 gram protein; 2.0 grams carbohydrates; 1.5 grams fat; 5 milligrams cholesterol; 65 milligrams sodium (without salting).

FARFALLINE AND LENTIL SOUP

Farfalline, which means "tiny butterflies," are one of the many pastas for soup created in Italy. Farfalline are shaped like miniature bows and make a very attractive presentation; however, if they're not available, any small pasta will do: anelli, shaped like rings, ditalini, which look like abbreviated elbow macaroni, or orzo, resembling grains of rice.

Served with slices of Tuscan bread this soup becomes a meal in a bowl.

2 teaspoons olive oil
1 onion, finely chopped
1 carrot, thinly sliced
1 large stalk celery, thinly sliced
4 plum tomatoes, diced
1/2 cup lentils, washed and picked over
5 cups low sodium beef broth, consomme, or stock
    Salt to taste
1/8 teaspoon hot red pepper flakes or to taste
1/2 cup farfalline (small pasta bows) or other small
    pasta

1. Heat oil in a soup pot. Add onion, carrot, and celery and cook over medium heat, stirring, for 2 minutes.

2. Reduce heat to low, add tomatoes to pot and cook, stirring occasionally, for 5 minutes. Add lentils, salt, and pepper flakes and stir to combine.

3. Raise heat slightly, add stock, and bring to a

simmer. Cover and cook, stirring occasionally and adding additional liquid if needed, for about 30 minutes or until lentils are almost tender.

4. Add farfalline and cook, uncovered, for 7 to 10 minutes or until al dente. Taste and correct seasoning, if necessary, before serving.

SERVES 4

Per serving: 285 calories; 13.0 grams protein; 47.0 grams carbohydrates; 5.3 grams fat; 7 milligrams cholesterol; 115 milligrams sodium (without salting).

CREAMY GREEN PEA–MACARONI SOUP WITH SMOKED CHICKEN

So what if the smoked chicken isn't the traditional ham hock—no one will resent the difference. But there is a difference in fat content in this streamlined version.

2 teaspoons olive oil
2 large shallots, minced
1 carrot, thinly sliced
1/4 pound smoked breast of chicken, cubed
4 cups Low Fat Chicken Stock (page 3) or canned low sodium broth
1/4 teaspoon thyme
1/2 cup small elbow macaroni
1 cup fresh or frozen and thawed green peas
1/2 cup low fat plain yogurt
Salt and freshly ground pepper to taste

1. Heat oil in a soup pot. Add shallots and carrot, and cook for 1 minute, stirring. Add chicken and cook for an additional minute.

2. Add stock and thyme and bring to a simmer. Add macaroni and peas and cook, uncovered, for about 10 minutes or until macaroni is al dente.

3. Gradually stir in yogurt as soup simmers. Season to taste with salt and pepper and cook soup for an additional 5 minutes or until ingredients are combined and heated through.

SERVES 4

Per serving: 235 calories; 13.5 grams protein; 33.0 grams carbohydrates; 5.5 grams fat; 20 milligrams cholesterol; 460 milligrams sodium (without salting).

TWO-FLAVOR CONSOMMÉ WITH PASTA AND PESTO

Using beef broth with the chicken stock adds body and flavor to this interesting and unusual soup. Pastina comes in a variety of shapes, including stars, tubes, and squares, and is also available in a spinach variety.

1 cup packed fresh basil leaves
1 clove garlic
1 tablespoon pignolias (pine nuts)
1 tablespoon olive oil
Salt and freshly ground pepper to taste
1 tablespoon grated low fat Parmesan cheese
2 cups low sodium beef broth, consomme, or stock
2 cups Low Fat Chicken Stock (page 3) or canned low sodium broth
1/2 cup pastina (tiny pasta)

1. Combine basil, garlic, nuts, oil, and seasonings in a food processor. Process until all ingredients are pureed. Spoon pesto into a small bowl. Stir in cheese and set aside.

2. Combine beef broth and chicken stock in a soup pot, cover, and bring to a simmer. Add pasta and cook until al dente.

3. Remove soup from heat and stir in pesto. Serve from a tureen or in individual heated soup bowls.

SERVES 4

Per serving: 185 calories; 6.5 grams protein; 24.0 grams carbohydrates; 7.0 grams fat; 6.0 milligrams cholesterol; 105 milligrams sodium (without salting).

FRESH TOMATO SOUP WITH ACINI DI PEPE

Acini di pepe are tiny bits of pasta, and well-named "grains of pepper," resembling grains of rice. If you have trouble finding this pasta shape, substitute orzo or another small pasta.

1½ pounds ripe plum tomatoes, chopped
  1 small onion, diced
  1 carrot, thinly sliced
  1 stalk celery, thinly sliced
  4 cups Low Fat Chicken Stock (page 3) or canned low sodium broth
 ½ teaspoon sugar
    Salt and freshly ground pepper to taste
 ½ cup acini di pepe
  1 tablespoon minced fresh Italian parsley

1. In a soup pot combine tomatoes, onion, carrot, celery, chicken stock, and sugar.

2. Cover and bring to a simmer. Cook for 30 minutes. Using a slotted spoon, remove solids from soup and puree in a food processor. Return puree to soup. Stir to combine and season to taste.

3. Return soup to a simmer and add acini di pepe. Cook until al dente, stirring occasionally.

4. Ladle soup into heated bowls and garnish with parsley before serving.

SERVES 4

Per serving: 185 calories; 6.5 grams protein; 34.0 grams carbohydrates; 2.5 grams fat; 5 milligrams cholesterol; 100 milligrams sodium (without salting).

HEARTY ORZO SOUP
WITH LAMB AND GREEN BEANS

Reminiscent of a soup I once enjoyed in Greece, this low fat, lemony orzo soup contains only a small quantity of lamb—less than an ounce per serving—yet it definitely has the richness and flavor of a "meaty" dish.

    3 ounces lean lamb, preferably from leg, cut into
        1/2-inch cubes
    2 cups water
    3 cups low sodium beef broth, consomme, or stock
    1/2 cup dry white wine
    1 tablespoon fresh lemon juice
    1 onion, chopped
    3 tablespoons chopped fresh Italian parsley
        Salt and freshly ground pepper to taste
    1 medium turnip, peeled and cut into 1/2-inch cubes
    1/4 pound green beans, trimmed and cut into 1-inch
        pieces
    1/2 cup orzo

1. Combine all ingredients, except turnip, green beans, and orzo, in a soup pot and bring to a boil. Cover, reduce heat to low and simmer gently for 45 minutes.

2. Add turnip to pot and simmer, covered, stirring occasionally, for an additional 20 minutes.

3. Add green beans and orzo and cook, uncovered, for about 10 minutes or until lamb, vegetables, and

orzo are tender. Taste and adjust seasoning, if necessary. Ladle into heated bowls and serve.

SERVES 4
Per serving: 190 calories; 10.0 grams protein; 31.0 grams carbohydrates; 2.7 grams fat; 18 milligrams cholesterol; 95 milligrams sodium (without salting).

JAPANESE NOODLE SOUP WITH SALMON AND SCALLIONS

This is my culinary homage to the classic Japanese film, *Tampopo*—a bright comedy about a female Japanese noodle-maker who strives to be the best. The wheat noodles (which are available in Asian markets, specialty stores, and some supermarkets) make a lovely, hearty, and satisfying dish, one that inspires me to do some heavy slurping—as is proper with Japanese noodles. I like to serve it with warm sake.

   2 cups fish stock or clam juice
   3 cups water
   6 ounces kishimen (Japanese wheat flour noodles)
³/₄ pound salmon fillet, poached and flaked, or canned
      red salmon, skin and bones removed
      Salt and freshly ground pepper to taste
   3 large scallions, white and tender greens, cut
      diagonally into bite-size pieces
   2 teaspoons orange or lemon zest

1. Combine clam juice and water in a soup pot and bring to a boil. Add the noodles and cook, with pot partially covered, for about 6 minutes or until noodles are softened.

2. Add salmon to pot and cook 1 to 2 minutes or until heated through. Season to taste with salt and pepper and remove from heat.

3. To serve, divide scallions among individual

heated shallow soup bowls. Ladle in soup with noodles and salmon, sprinkle with zest, and serve immediately.

SERVES 4
Per serving: 285 calories; 22.0 grams protein; 34.5 grams carbohydrates; 6.0 grams fat; 47 milligrams cholesterol; 850 milligrams sodium (without salting).

PUMPKIN-RICE SOUP
WITH GINGER

Fresh or canned pumpkin can be used in this soup, but if you opt for the canned, use the low sodium, sugar free variety. Or, if you prefer, you can substitute butternut squash for the pumpkin.

2 teaspoons olive oil
1 small onion, diced
2 cups peeled, seeded, and cubed fresh pumpkin
5 cups Low Fat Chicken Stock (page 3) or canned low sodium broth
2 teaspoons grated fresh ginger
1/4 teaspoon ground cardamom
1/4 cup rice
Salt and freshly ground pepper to taste
1/4 cup minced fresh chives

1. Heat olive oil in a soup pot. Add onion and cook, stirring, for 2 minutes.

2. Add all remaining ingredients, except salt, pepper, and chives. Stir to combine and bring to a simmer. Cover and cook for about 20 minutes or until pumpkin and rice are tender.

3. Season to taste and serve garnished with chives.

SERVES 4

Per serving: 120 calories; 3.0 grams protein; 17.5 grams carbohydrates; 4.5 grams fat; 7 milligrams cholesterol; 85 milligrams sodium (without salting).

BROWN RICE AND BEAN CHOWDER WITH CARROT CURLS

To save on the cooking time, this soup can be made using canned white beans, but drain and rinse them well before using to remove excess salt.

 $^1/_2$ cup Great Northern or white beans, rinsed and drained
 1 teaspoon olive oil
 2 shallots, minced
 1 clove garlic, pressed
 $^1/_2$ cup brown rice
 6 cups Low Fat Chicken Stock (page 3) or canned low sodium broth
 $^1/_4$ teaspoon dried thyme
    Salt and freshly ground pepper to taste
 1 medium carrot
    Ice water

1. Combine beans with enough water to amply cover in a large saucepan. Bring to a boil and cook for 2 minutes. Cover, remove from heat, and let stand for 1 hour.

2. Drain beans. Add enough fresh water to amply cover beans and cook, covered, 45 minutes to $1^1/_2$ hours or until tender. (Cooking time will depend on the age of the beans.) Drain beans and set aside.

3. While beans cook, heat oil in a large soup pot. Add shallots and garlic and cook, stirring, for 2 min-

utes. Add rice and cook, stirring, for an additional minute. Add stock and thyme, cover, and cook about 30 minutes or until rice is tender. Remove from heat.

4. Place half of cooked beans in a food processor. Add 1 cup of liquid from soup and puree. Add bean puree and remaining beans to soup. Stir and bring to a simmer. Add salt and pepper to taste and cook for 10 minutes.

5. While soup heats make carrot curls by running a vegetable peeler lengthwise down the carrot, then place in a bowl of ice water until ready to use. Drain well before using.

6. Serve soup from a tureen or ladle into individual heated bowls. Garnish with carrot curls before serving.

Serves 6

Per serving: 150 calories; 5.5 grams protein; 26.0 grams carbohydrates; 2.8 grams fat; 5 milligrams cholesterol; 75 milligrams sodium (without salting).

CURRIED CAULIFLOWER-RICE SOUP WITH PEAR

If the aroma doesn't woo you, the flavor will because the light curry taste complements both the rice and the fruit. Apples are also good in this soup. Pair it with a good Indian-style bread or with toasted pita points.

2 teaspoons vegetable oil
1 small onion, finely chopped
2 teaspoons grated peeled ginger
1 pear, peeled, cored, and diced
2 cups cauliflower florets
4 cups Low Fat Chicken Stock (page 3) or canned low sodium broth
1 teaspoon curry powder or to taste
Pinch cayenne pepper or to taste
1/4 cup basmati rice, rinsed and drained

1. Heat vegetable oil in a soup pot. Add onion, ginger, pear, and cauliflower, and cook, stirring, for 3 minutes.

2. Add stock, curry, and cayenne pepper to pot and bring to a simmer. Cover and cook for 10 minutes.

3. Remove soup from heat. Spoon 1 cup of solids from soup into a food processor and puree. Return puree to soup pot.

4. Add rice to soup, stir, and bring back to a sim-

mer. Cover and cook for about 20 minutes or until rice is tender.

SERVES 4

Per serving: 135 calories; 3.0 grams protein; 21.5 grams carbohydrates; 4.3 grams fat; 5 milligrams cholesterol; 75 milligrams sodium (without salting).

WILD RICE, BARLEY,
AND MUSHROOM CHOWDER

This soul-stirring soup is the perfect picker-upper on even the darkest, dreariest days. For a slightly sweet taste, substitute parsnip for the turnip.

   2 teaspoons olive oil
   1 small onion, diced
   1 small carrot, thinly sliced
   1 small turnip, diced
   1 medium red jacket potato, diced
   1/4 pound mushrooms, wiped clean and thinly sliced
   1 clove garlic, pressed
   1/4 cup wild rice
   1/4 cup barley
   6 cups Low Fat Chicken Stock (page 3) or canned low
      sodium broth
      Salt and freshly ground pepper to taste
   2 tablespoons minced fresh parsley

1. Heat oil in a soup pot. Add onion, carrot, turnip, and potato, and cook over low heat, stirring occasionally, for 3 minutes.

2. Add mushrooms and garlic to pot and cook, stirring frequently, for 2 minutes.

3. Add wild rice, barley, and stock to pot and stir to combine. Bring to a simmer, cover, and cook for about 45 minutes or until wild rice and barley are tender.

4. Season to taste with salt and pepper and serve garnished with parsley.

Serves 6
Per serving: 125 calories; 4.0 grams protein; 19.5 grams carbohydrates; 4.3 grams fat; 5 milligrams cholesterol; 90 milligrams sodium (without salting).

BARLEY AND LEEK SOUP
WITH PROSCIUTTO

This hearty soup will be appreciated on a cold wintry day. The prosciutto is added to flavor the soup; if you prefer, you can substitute smoked turkey or chicken.

2 teaspoons vegetable oil
2 leeks, white and tender greens, rinsed and chopped
2 cloves garlic, chopped
1 large carrot, chopped
1 large stalk celery, chopped
1 ounce prosciutto, preferably in one piece, chopped
$\frac{1}{2}$ teaspoon dried marjoram
$\frac{1}{2}$ teaspoon dried basil
   Salt and freshly ground pepper to taste
$\frac{1}{2}$ cup pearl barley
4 cups beef broth, consomme, or stock, homemade or canned
1 large potato, peeled and diced

1. Heat oil in a soup pot. Add all remaining ingredients, except barley, broth, and potato and cook over medium heat for 5 minutes, stirring frequently.

2. Add barley and broth to pot. Reduce heat to low, cover, and simmer gently for 1 hour.

3. Add potato to pot and continue to simmer for an additional 10 minutes or until potato is tender.

SERVES 4

Per serving: 245 calories; 7.5 grams protein; 41.5 grams carbohydrates; 6.0 grams fat; 5 milligrams cholesterol; 230 milligrams sodium (without salting).

APPETIZERS
AND
STARTERS

BROAD NOODLES
WITH GARLIC AND CHICKPEAS

Today, the traditional broad egg noodles may be purchased egg-less. If you're watching your cholesterol the noodles without eggs will do just fine in this recipe.

 ¹/₂ cup cooked or canned (rinsed and drained)
       chickpeas
1¹/₂ cups Low Fat Chicken Stock (page 3) or canned low
       sodium broth
  2 cloves garlic, quartered
  2 teaspoons olive oil
  1 shallot, minced
    Salt and freshly ground pepper to taste
 ¹/₄ pound broad noodles
  8 fresh basil leaves

1. Combine ¹/₄ cup chickpeas, ¹/₂ cup stock, and garlic in a food processor and puree coarsely. Set aside.

2. Heat oil in a large skillet. Sauté shallot for 2 minutes, stirring.

3. Add chickpea puree, remainder of chickpeas, and remainder of stock to skillet. Cover and cook over low heat for 5 minutes. Season to taste with salt and pepper and set aside.

4. Cook noodles in a large pot full of boiling water until al dente. (Noodles cook more quickly than other pastas, be careful not to overcook.)

5. Drain noodles and add to skillet with chickpeas. Toss to combine ingredients and cook until just heated through.

6. To serve, mound noodles and chickpeas onto plates and top each serving with 2 basil leaves.

SERVES 4

Per serving: 175 calories; 6.5 grams protein; 27.0 grams carbohydrates; 4.5 grams fat; 29 milligrams cholesterol; 35 milligrams sodium (without salting).

CAULIFLOWER AND CARROTS OVER THIN SPAGHETTI

Cauliflower is a crucifer, a member of the family of vegetables—which includes broccoli and cabbage—that is thought may be an anticancer agent. It is definitely nutritious and extremely low in fat and calories, so fill up without guilt.

½ small head cauliflower (about ½ pound), trimmed
1 tablespoon cider vinegar
2 teaspoons olive oil
1 clove garlic, pressed
½ cup Low Fat Chicken Stock (page 3) or canned low sodium broth
¼ pound thin spaghetti
Salt and freshly ground pepper to taste
1 carrot, grated

1. Cover and cook cauliflower in a large saucepan full of boiling water to which cider vinegar has been added for about 10 minutes or until cauliflower is tender. Drain and let cool slightly.

2. When cauliflower is cool enough to handle, separate into florets and set aside.

3. Heat oil in a large nonstick skillet. Add garlic and sauté for 1 minute, stirring. Add stock and bring to a simmer. Add cauliflower florets to skillet and toss to combine. Remove from heat.

4. Cook spaghetti in a large pot full of boiling water (salted, if desired) until al dente. Drain and add

to cauliflower in skillet. Toss to combine, season to taste, and heat through.

5. Transfer ingredients from skillet to a heated platter and top with grated carrot before serving.

SERVES 4
Per serving: 145 calories; 4.5 grams protein; 24.5 grams carbohydrates; 3.0 grams fat; 1 milligram cholesterol; 20 milligrams sodium (without salting).

PESTO OVER LASAGNA
NOODLES

Lasagna noodles can be used in more than one way. Rather than layering them, here's a recipe that uses lasagna as a base for basil and parsley pesto.

1 cup packed fresh basil leaves
1/4 cup packed fresh parsley leaves
1 clove garlic
2 teaspoons pignolias (pine nuts)
2 teaspoons olive oil
   Salt and freshly ground pepper to taste
1 tablespoon grated low fat Parmesan cheese
4 lasagna noodles

1. Combine basil, parsley, garlic, nuts, oil, and salt and pepper in a food processor. Process until ingredients are pureed. Spoon pesto into a bowl, stir in cheese, and set aside.

2. In a large saucepan full of boiling water (salted, if desired) cook lasagna noodles until al dente. As pasta cooks add 3 tablespoons of the pasta water to the pesto sauce and mix well.

3. Drain lasagna noodles and place, folded or cut in half, on heated dishes. Spoon equal amounts of pesto over each lasagna noodle and serve at once.

SERVES 4

Per serving: 130 calories; 5.0 grams protein; 18.5 grams carbohydrates; 4.0 grams fat; 1 milligram cholesterol; 40 milligrams sodium (without salting).

MUSHROOM AND CORN PASTA ROLLS IN BÉCHAMEL SAUCE

Here, lasagna noodles are rolled around a delicious filling of mushrooms and corn, topped with light béchamel sauce, and baked until bubbling.

¼ cup Low Fat Chicken Stock (page 3) or canned low sodium broth
¾ pound mushrooms, wiped clean and thinly sliced
½ cup fresh white corn kernels, or frozen and thawed
Pinch cayenne pepper or to taste
Salt to taste
8 lasagna noodles

BÉCHAMEL SAUCE
1 teaspoon olive oil
¼ cup chopped fresh chives
¼ cup Low Fat Chicken Stock (page 3) or canned low sodium broth
1½ tablespoons fine flour
1 cup low fat (1%) milk
Salt and freshly ground white pepper to taste
Vegetable oil cooking spray

1. Preheat oven to 350° F.
2. Combine stock, mushrooms, corn, cayenne, and salt in a medium saucepan. Cover and cook over medium heat for about 8 minutes or until mushrooms and corn are tender. Season to taste and set aside.

3. Cook lasagna noodles in a large pot full of boiling water (salted, if desired) until al dente. Drain pasta and place on a clean dishcloth. Pat dry.

4. Prepare béchamel sauce while pasta cooks. Heat oil in a small heavy saucepan. Add chives and stock, and cook, stirring, for 1 minute. Add flour and stir to combine. Cook over very low heat, stirring, for 2 minutes. Add milk and continue to cook over low heat, stirring, until sauce thickens. Season with salt and pepper and remove from heat.

5. Add $1/3$ of béchamel sauce to mushroom mixture, stir to combine and set aside.

6. Transfer lasagna to a board or other flat surface. Spoon $1/8$ of mushroom mixture on a strip of lasagna and roll. Repeat with remaining mushroom mixture and lasagna.

7. Place lasagna rolls, seam-side down, in a nonstick baking pan or casserole lightly coated with vegetable oil spray. Rolls should be touching. Spoon on remaining béchamel sauce, cover pan with foil, and bake for 25 minutes. Remove foil and bake an additional 5 to 10 minutes or until bubbly. Serve immediately.

SERVES 8

Per serving: 125 calories; 5.0 grams protein; 22.5 grams carbohydrates; 1.7 grams fat; 2 milligrams cholesterol; 35 milligrams sodium (without salting).

FETTUCCINE WITH JALAPEÑO PEPPER, DRIED TOMATOES, AND GARLIC

The tomatoes and garlic take some of the heat from the jalapeños without extinguishing their fire. Linguine or spinach-flavored fettuccine could be used instead of the regular fettuccine.

 1/4 cup no-salt-added dried tomatoes
  2 teaspoons olive oil
  1 small jalapeño pepper, trimmed and finely chopped
  4 cloves garlic, pressed
  4 plum tomatoes, diced
    Salt and freshly ground pepper to taste
 1/4 pound fettuccine

1. Cover tomatoes with boiling water and let stand 5 minutes. Drain and mince.

2. Heat oil in a large nonstick skillet. Add tomatoes, jalapeño pepper, and garlic. Cook, stirring, for 3 minutes.

3. Add plum tomatoes to skillet. Cover and cook over low heat for 15 minutes. Season to taste.

4. While sauce simmers, cook fettucine in a large pot full of boiling water (salted, if desired) until al dente. Drain.

5. Add fettuccine to skillet. Heat through and toss to combine ingredients. Transfer to a large heated bowl or individual plates and serve.

SERVES 4

Per serving: 170 calories; 5.0 grams protein; 30.0 grams carbohydrates; 3.3 grams fat; 0 milligrams cholesterol; 20 milligrams sodium (without salting).

FUSILLI WITH SAUSAGE AND ROASTED PEPPER

Roasting intensifies the flavor of the pepper (or most vegetables, for that matter) and gives this sauce its real substance. The sausage and fennel seeds are brilliant supporting players.

1 large red bell pepper
1/4 pound fusilli (corkscrew) pasta
2 teaspoons olive oil
3 ounces Italian-style turkey sausage, thinly sliced
1/2 teaspoon ground fennel seeds
   Salt and freshly ground pepper to taste
1/4 cup chopped fresh basil

1. Preheat oven to broil.
2. Place a sheet of foil on a broiling pan. Place pepper on foil and broil. Turn pepper from side to side until skin is charred.
3. Place pepper in a paper bag and allow to cool. Peel and scrape off charred skin. Cut pepper into thin slices and set aside.
4. While pepper broils, cook pasta in a large pot full of boiling water (salted, if desired) until al dente. Drain and set aside.
5. Heat oil in a large nonstick skillet. Add sausage and cook over medium heat until brown on all sides and cooked through. Add pepper slices and fennel seeds.
6. Add pasta to skillet. Season to taste and toss to

combine ingredients. Heat through and transfer to heated dishes. Garnish with basil and serve.

SERVES 4

Per serving: 175 calories; 7.5 grams protein; 23.5 grams carbohydrates; 5.8 grams fat; 23 milligrams cholesterol; 150 milligrams sodium (without salting).

WATERCRESS AND RICOTTA WONTON RAVIOLI

Although there's no substitute for ravioli made from scratch, preparing it with fresh or frozen wonton skins or wrappers (which are readily available at supermarkets everywhere) saves a good deal of time and work.

For this starter, I've filled the wonton skins with a mixture of watercress and ricotta flavored with shallots and herbs. I've also added watercress, plus a touch of garlic and a sprinkling of Parmesan to the tomato sauce dressing. All in all, a sensational way to start a meal; this one is guaranteed to garner compliments.

    1 cup packed watercress
  1/2 cup low fat ricotta cheese
    2 shallots, finely minced
    1 clove garlic, pressed
  1/4 teaspoon each: dried basil, marjoram, and thyme, or
        to taste
      Salt and freshly ground pepper to taste
      Egg substitute equal to 1 egg
   24 wonton wrappers, fresh or frozen and thawed
    1 cup canned no-salt-added tomato sauce
    4 teaspoons grated low fat Parmesan cheese

1. Blanch watercress in boiling water for 1 minute. Drain and set aside.

2. In a small bowl, combine half of the watercress

with ricotta, shallots, garlic, herbs, salt and pepper, and egg substitute. Stir to blend ingredients.

3. Place wonton wrappers on a platter and cover with a damp, clean kitchen towel. Lightly flour a work area and lay one wrapper on floured surface. (Keep remaining wonton wrappers covered as they dry out quickly.)

4. Place about a tablespoon of watercress-ricotta mixture in the center of wrapper, moisten the edges with water and lay a second wrapper on top, pushing from filling outward to remove as much air as possible. Seal edges with light pressure and trim with a knife or cookie cutter into a square or an attractive shape, if desired. Place the finished ravioli to dry slightly on paper towels. Continue until you have made 12 ravioli.

5. In a small saucepan, combine tomato sauce with remaining watercress, and season to taste with salt and pepper if desired. Let simmer, stirring occasionally, over low heat until needed.

6. Bring a large pot of water to a slow boil (do not let water boil too rapidly or ravioli might fall apart). Add ravioli, 3 or 4 at a time, and cook gently for about 4 minutes or until ravioli rise to the surface. Remove with a slotted spoon to a warm bowl until they are all cooked.

7. Place 3 ravioli in center of individual heated bowls or plates. Spoon sauce over ravioli, sprinkle each with a teaspoon of Parmesan, and serve.

SERVES 4

Per serving: 270 calories; 13.0 grams protein; 49.5 grams carbohydrates; 3.0 grams fat; 9 milligrams cholesterol; 500 milligrams sodium (without salting).

CRABMEAT SUI MAI DUMPLINGS

"Sui mai" (pronounced shoo-my) is one of the most popular Cantonese "dim sum" dishes. In Canton province dim sum refers to the tasty tidbits served in teahouses for breakfast and lunch, while in other parts of China it means snack food.

Prepare this sui mai in advance and resteam for terrific hors d'oeuvres. Instead of the hot mustard or chili pepper paste, you may want to try it with my Asian Dipping Sauce (page 46) on the side.

    3 dried shiitake or Chinese mushrooms
    3 ounces very lean ground turkey or chicken
    1 tablespoon dry sherry, sake, or Chinese Shao-sing
        wine
    Freshly ground white pepper to taste
    2 teaspoons low sodium soy sauce
    1/2 tablespoon cornstarch
    3 ounces crabmeat, fresh or frozen and thawed, picked
        over
    1 tablespoon chopped scallions
    1/4 cup minced water chestnuts or bamboo shoots
    1 teaspoon sesame oil
    24 wonton wrappers, fresh or frozen and thawed, cut
        into 3-inch rounds
    Lettuce leaves
    Hot Asian mustard or chili pepper paste

1. Soak mushrooms in about 1/2 cup hot water for 30 minutes. Remove stems and cut into thin (julienne) slices. Set aside.

2. Combine turkey or chicken, wine, pepper, soy sauce, and cornstarch in a large bowl and blend well. Add mushrooms, crabmeat, scallions, water chestnuts, and sesame oil and mix until ingredients are thoroughly combined.

3. Spoon about 2 teaspoons of the filling in the middle of each wonton wrapper. With fingertips, pucker the wrapper around stuffing, leaving tops open, making the sui mai look like a filled, puckered cup. Flatten the bottoms by gently tapping the dumplings on the work surface.

4. Place dumplings in a large Asian steamer on a layer of lettuce leaves (or on a plate lightly coated with vegetable spray) and steam for 10 minutes. Serve hot on individual plates immediately with a tiny bit of mustard or chili paste on the side.

SERVES 6
Per serving: 175 calories; 10.0 grams protein; 31.5 grams carbohydrates; 1.6 grams fat; 14 milligrams cholesterol; 535 milligrams sodium (without salting).

APPETIZER WONTONS
WITH ASIAN DIPPING SAUCE

Instead of boiling in stock, these wontons may also be fried in batches—using a nonstick skillet with a thin film of vegetable oil spray. For a hearty soup, I like to simmer these in broth and add some chopped scallion, mustard greens, and shredded cooked chicken.

1/2 pound very lean ground turkey, chicken, or pork tenderloin
2 teaspoons cornstarch
1 tablespoon low sodium soy sauce
2 teaspoons dry sherry (not cooking wine)
1/2 teaspoon sesame oil
1 1/2 teaspoons vegetable oil
Salt and freshly ground pepper to taste
4 small shrimp, cooked and finely chopped
1 egg white
4 scallions, white and tender greens, finely chopped
6 water chestnuts, finely chopped
40 wonton wrappers, fresh or frozen and thawed
2 cups Low Fat Chicken Stock (page 3) or canned low sodium broth

ASIAN DIPPING SAUCE
3 tablespoons rice wine vinegar
2 tablespoons low sodium soy sauce
1 teaspoon sesame oil
1 tablespoon finely minced scallions

1 tablespoon finely minced chopped fresh parsley or
   cilantro

1. Combine turkey, cornstarch, soy sauce, sherry, and sesame oil. Mix well and set aside.
2. Heat oil in a large nonstick skillet. Add turkey mixture and cook, stirring and breaking up clumps, for 4 to 5 minutes or until meat is cooked through.
3. Using a slotted spoon, transfer turkey mixture from skillet to a large bowl. Add all remaining ingredients, except wonton wrappers and stock and mix until filling is thoroughly blended.
4. Place about 1 teaspoon of filling in center of a wonton wrapper, keeping unused wrappers covered with a clean damp cloth. Moisten half of wrapper edge with water and fold over wrapper to form a triangle. Press firmly around edges to seal. Moisten left tip of triangle, bring right tip to meet it, and press tips together. Repeat until all wonton wrappers are used.
5. Place stock in a medium saucepan and bring to a slow boil. Simmer wontons, a few at a time, for 4 to 5 minutes or until they rise to surface. Remove with slotted spoon and keep warm.
6. While wontons cook, combine ingredients for Asian Dipping Sauce in a small bowl. Let stand at room temperature until needed.
7. Serve wontons with dipping sauce on the side.

SERVES 10
Per serving: 185 calories; 10.0 grams protein; 30.5 grams carbohydrates; 3.0 grams fat; 15 milligrams cholesterol; 600 milligrams sodium (without salting).

TOMATOES STUFFED
WITH RICE AND SEA SCALLOPS

Fresh sweet sea scallops, always available during tomato season, add panache to humdrum tomato surprise. This dish works equally well with shrimp.

    1 cup rice
 1¹/₂ cups water
   ¹/₄ teaspoon ground turmeric
       Pinch cayenne pepper or to taste
       Salt to taste
     4 medium tomatoes
     4 large sea scallops
     1 teaspoon olive oil
     1 teaspoon freshly ground pepper

1. Combine rice, water, turmeric, cayenne pepper, and salt in a heavy saucepan with a lid. Cover and bring to a boil. Lower heat to a simmer and cook for about 15 minutes or until rice is tender and liquid is absorbed. If rice is not tender and water has been absorbed add more water, 2 tablespoons at a time. Remove rice from heat and allow to return to room temperature. Add salt to taste.

2. While rice cooks, cut a slice from the top of each tomato and reserve slice. Using a spoon scoop out seeds and most of pulp from each tomato. Salt to taste and invert on a plate, allowing tomatoes to drain for 20 minutes.

3. Rinse scallops and pat dry. Cut each scallop in half, horizontally.

4. Heat oil in a medium nonstick skillet. When oil is very hot add scallops and cook for 1 minute on each side, browning lightly. Drain on paper towel and season both sides with pepper. Reserve.

5. Turn tomatoes right-side up and spoon rice into tomatoes, allowing rice to come just below top of each tomato. Carefully place two scallop slices over rice on each tomato and top with reserved tomato slice to create a cap. Serve at room temperature or chilled.

SERVES 4

Per serving: 220 calories; 7.0 grams protein; 43.5 grams carbohydrates; 2.0 grams fat; 5 milligrams cholesterol; 40 milligrams sodium (without salting).

BELL PEPPERS STUFFED WITH BASMATI RICE AND PEAS

Isn't it nice to know that you don't have to give up some of your favorite appetizers, even though you're eating a lighter diet? The rice, peas, and slightly crunchy pepper add texture, color, and flavor without adding fat.

2 large bell peppers (green, red, yellow, or
    combination)
2 cups Low Fat Chicken Stock (page 3) or canned low
    sodium broth
1 cup basmati rice, rinsed and drained
1/2 cup fresh or frozen and thawed green peas
1/4 teaspoon ground cumin
    Salt and freshly ground pepper to taste
1 tablespoon minced fresh cilantro
3/4 cup canned no-salt-added tomato sauce, heated

1. Cut bell peppers in half, lengthwise, core, and seed.

2. Blanch pepper halves in a large pot full of boiling water for 3 to 5 minutes, or until just tender. Invert on paper towels to drain.

3. Bring stock to a boil in a large saucepan. Add rice, stir, and return to a boil. Cover and reduce heat to a simmer. Cook rice for 15 minutes.

4. Add peas to rice. Cover and cook for an additional 5 to 8 minutes or until rice is tender and liquid

has been absorbed. Remove from heat. Fluff rice with a fork and let stand, covered, for 5 minutes.

5. Add cumin, salt, pepper, and ½ tablespoon cilantro to rice. Mix to combine ingredients.

6. Place pepper halves, cut-side up, on a heated platter. Stuff pepper halves with rice mixture. Spoon equal amounts of hot tomato sauce over each pepper half, sprinkle with remaining cilantro, and serve.

SERVES 4

Per serving: 220 calories; 5.5 grams protein; 46.0 grams carbohydrates; 1.5 grams fat; 3 milligrams cholesterol; 50 milligrams sodium (without salting).

RICE AND SEAFOOD QUICHE

Quiche, which is traditionally made with a savory custard consisting of eggs, cream, cheese, and various other ingredients, may be delicious but it's definitely not in keeping with a reduced-fat diet. For this quiche, I've substituted low fat ingredients and the result is equally delicious—and it has a total fat content you can definitely live with.

>   Vegetable oil cooking spray
>   2 cups cooked rice, cooled to room temperature
>   3 ounces shrimp, shelled, deveined, cooked, and diced
>   3 ounces bay scallops, cooked and diced
>   4 scallions, white and tender greens, finely sliced
>   1 small green bell pepper, finely diced
> 1 1/2 tablespoons diced pimientos
>   1/2 teaspoon paprika or to taste
>   Salt to taste
>   1/2 cup shredded low fat Swiss cheese (about 2 ounces)
>   2/3 cup low fat (1%) milk
>   Egg substitute equal to 3 eggs

1. Preheat oven to 350° F. Coat a 10-inch pie plate or ovenproof casserole with cooking spray and set aside.

2. In a large bowl, combine all ingredients, except milk and egg substitute. Toss to blend. Add milk and egg substitute and stir until ingredients are thoroughly blended.

3. Spoon rice-shrimp mixture into prepared pan or

casserole and bake for about 30 minutes or until a knife inserted in center comes out clean.

4. Let stand 2 minutes before serving.

SERVES 4

Per serving: 305 calories; 20.5 grams protein; 42.5 grams carbohydrates; 6.0 grams fat; 54 milligrams cholesterol; 170 milligrams sodium (without salting).

SPICY COUSCOUS WITH SALSA

Is couscous a grain or a pasta? There is a difference of opinion. One food authority describes it as cracked, uncooked wheat, resembling semolina, while another says it's a pasta made by rolling bits of durum wheat in flour. Both semolina and durum wheat are ingredients in the flour that goes into pasta—so however you choose to define couscous, it makes good eating.

Regular couscous requires lengthy cooking time, and is usually prepared in a special steamer. However, a quick-cooking couscous is now available in most supermarkets, thus making the preparation of this interesting grain/pasta starter much easier.

  2 teaspoons olive oil
  1 small onion, diced
  2 cloves garlic, pressed
  2 shallots, minced
1½ cups Low Fat Chicken Stock (page 3) or canned low
       sodium broth
  ½ teaspoon ground cumin
    Pinch cayenne pepper
  1 cup quick-cooking couscous
  3 plum tomatoes, finely chopped
  2 teaspoons hot pepper sauce or to taste
    Salt and freshly ground pepper to taste

1. Heat olive oil in a large nonstick saucepan or deep skillet. Add onion, garlic, and shallots and cook, stirring, for 2 minutes.

2. Add stock, cumin, and cayenne to saucepan and bring to a boil. Add couscous, cover and cook for 2 minutes. Remove from heat and let stand for 5 to 10 minutes, or until couscous is tender.

3. Meanwhile, combine tomatoes and hot pepper sauce in a small bowl. Mix well and set aside.

4. When couscous is tender, season to taste with salt and pepper and mound in the center of individual dishes. Top each with salsa and serve.

SERVES 6
Per serving: 155 calories; 5.0 grams protein; 29.0 grams carbohydrates; 2.2 grams fat; 2 milligrams cholesterol; 55 milligrams sodium (without salting).

TABBOULEH WITH FENNEL IN LETTUCE ROLLS

Tabbouleh, a great favorite in most Middle Eastern countries, is prepared with bulgur. Bulgur is cracked wheat that has been cooked and dried, and has been currently renamed in many stores as "wheat berries." Fine-grained bulgur needs no additional cooking, though it does have to be rehydrated by soaking. Larger-grained bulgur used in soups, stuffings, and pilafs is cooked and expands as it absorbs liquid.

1/2 cup fine bulgur
4 cups water
1/2 cup thinly sliced fennel
2 scallions, white and tender greens, thinly sliced
2 plum tomatoes, diced
1/4 cup minced fresh parsley
1 tablespoon dried crumbled mint
2 tablespoons fresh lemon juice
1 tablespoon olive oil
Salt and freshly ground pepper to taste
Lettuce leaves

1. Combine bulgur and water in a large bowl. Allow bulgur to soak for about 30 minutes. Drain and transfer to a colander that has been lined with a clean dishcloth. Draw cloth tightly together and squeeze out water. Transfer bulgur to another large bowl.

2. Add fennel, scallions, tomatoes, parsley, and mint to bulgur and mix to combine ingredients.

3. Combine lemon juice and oil in a small, screw-top jar. Shake well, and pour slowly over bulgur, mixing thoroughly. Season to taste.

4. Pile bulgur in a mound in the center of a serving platter and surround with lettuce leaves. Serve, allowing each person to roll tabbouleh in the lettuce leaves.

SERVES 4

Per serving: 110 calories; 3.0 grams protein; 17.0 grams carbohydrates; 4.0 grams fat; 0 milligrams cholesterol; 25 milligrams sodium (without salting).

SALADS

TRICOLORED PASTA–TUNA SALAD WITH APPLE AND CURRANTS

A tasty, creamy dressing made lower in fat by substituting low fat mayo and plain yogurt for straight, full-strength mayonnaise alone. The tart sweetness of apples and dried currants makes this any-weather pasta and tuna salad truly memorable.

1/2 pound tricolored pasta spirals or twists
2 tablespoons low fat mayonnaise
2 tablespoons low fat plain yogurt
1 tablespoon fresh lemon juice
1 tablespoon chopped fresh parsley or 1/2 tablespoon
   dried
1/2 teaspoon dry mustard
1/4 teaspoon dried tarragon
   Salt and freshly ground pepper to taste
2 stalks celery, diced
1/4 cup dried currants
1 large Granny Smith or other tart apple, cored and
   cubed
1 can (6 1/8 ounces) chunk light tuna in water

1. Cook pasta in a large pot full of boiling water (salted, if desired) until al dente. Drain, transfer to a large bowl, and set aside to cool.
2. Combine mayonnaise, yogurt, lemon juice, parsley, mustard, tarragon, and salt and pepper in a

small bowl. Stir until ingredients are thoroughly combined. Set aside.

3. Add all remaining ingredients to pasta in bowl. Toss lightly.

4. Spoon on mayonnaise dressing and toss again until all ingredients are blended and coated with dressing. Transfer to a platter or individual dishes and serve.

SERVES 4

Per serving: 340 calories; 19.0 grams protein; 55.5 grams carbohydrates; 4.2 grams fat; 15 milligrams cholesterol; 225 milligrams sodium (without salting).

BOWS WITH SWEET PEPPERS AND HERB POTPOURRI

Fresh herbs work best for this dish, but dried (use approximately half the amount) can be used in a pinch. If garlic chives (grown from garlic bulbs) are unavailable, use the regular or onion chives.

1/2 pound farfalle (pasta bows)
1/2 small yellow bell pepper, finely chopped
1/2 small red bell pepper, finely chopped
1/2 small green bell pepper, finely chopped
2 tablespoons chopped fresh basil
2 tablespoons chopped fresh parsley
1 tablespoon chopped garlic chives
2 tablespoons vegetable or chicken broth
1 tablespoon olive oil
  Pinch hot red pepper flakes or to taste
  Salt to taste

1. Cook pasta in a large pot full of boiling water (salted, if desired) until al dente. Drain and set aside to cool.

2. Combine all remaining ingredients in a large bowl and mix until thoroughly combined.

3. Transfer pasta to a serving bowl. Spoon pepper-herb mixture over pasta and mix well. Taste and correct seasoning if necessary. Serve at room temperature or chilled.

SERVES 4

Per serving: 250 calories; 7.5 grams protein; 43.5 grams carbohydrates; 4.6 grams fat; 0 milligrams cholesterol; 10 milligrams sodium (without salting).

BOWS AND BEANS
WITH RED ONIONS

The Italians have long known the sensual pleasure pasta and bean dishes leave in the mouth. *Pasta e fagioli*, the thick soup composed primarily of macaroni and beans, comes immediately to mind. This unusual vegetarian salad produces the same kind of dreamy satisfaction. It's best served slightly warm or at room temperature.

1/2 pound farfalle (pasta bows)
1/2 cup cooked pinto or kidney beans
1 large red onion, cut in half and thinly sliced
1/4 cup canned low sodium tomato juice
2 teaspoons olive oil
1 teaspoon fresh lemon juice
1/2 teaspoon dried basil or parsley
1/4 teaspoon dried thyme
Salt and freshly ground pepper to taste

1. Cook pasta in a large pot full of boiling water (salted, if desired) until al dente. Drain and transfer to a large bowl.

2. Add beans and onions to pasta.

3. Combine all remaining ingredients in a screw-top jar. Close tightly and shake until thoroughly combined.

4. Spoon dressing over pasta and beans, toss to combine all ingredients, and serve.

Per serving: 285 calories; 10.0 grams protein; 52.5 grams carbohydrates; 3.5 grams fat; 0 milligrams cholesterol; 10 milligrams sodium (without salting).

PENNE SALAD WITH SNOW PEAS, HAM, AND CHEESE IN DIJON DRESSING

Long gone are the days when I could (or would) order and happily devour a chef's salad and still feel good about myself for having done so, for the standard version contains both ham and roast beef, Swiss cheese, sliced hard-cooked eggs, and turkey, all cut into strips. Shards of lettuce and tomato and a blanket of mayonnaise-y Russian or Thousand Island dressing complete the dish. Of course time—and chefs—change, as do our needs. And so I've devised this chef-style salad with lower-in-fat ingredients and a dynamite Dijon/balsamic vinaigrette to still guilt, awaken the taste buds, and satisfy hunger pangs. I like to offer this salad as a buffet selection.

  1 clove garlic, pressed
  $^1/_3$ cup low fat plain yogurt
  1 tablespoon balsamic vinegar
  2 teaspoons olive oil
  2 teaspoons Dijon mustard
  1 teaspoon minced fresh Italian parsley
    Salt and freshly ground pepper to taste
  $^1/_2$ pound penne
  $1^1/_2$ cups fresh snow peas
  1 ounce low fat ham, shredded
  1 ounce Jarlsberg or Swiss cheese, shredded

1. Combine garlic, yogurt, vinegar, oil, mustard, parsley, and salt and pepper in a screw-top jar. Close tightly and shake until combined. Set aside.

2. Cook pasta in a large pot full of boiling water (salted, if desired) until al dente. Drain and place in a large bowl.

3. While pasta cooks, blanch snow peas in boiling water for 1 minute. Drain and rinse under cold water.

4. Add snow peas, ham, and cheese to pasta in bowl. Spoon dressing over all and toss to combine. Correct seasoning, if necessary, transfer to a platter or individual dishes, and serve.

SERVES 4

Per serving: 295 calories; 12.0 grams protein; 47.5 grams carbohydrates; 5.8 grams fat; 8 milligrams cholesterol; 160 milligrams sodium (without salting).

PASTA SHELLS WITH SEAFOOD, PEPPERS, AND PEARL TOMATOES

Pearl tomatoes are seasonal and may be difficult to find; if necessary substitute the tiniest cherry tomatoes or cut the larger ones in half before garnishing this lovely salad.

1/4 cup vegetable or chicken broth
2 teaspoons olive oil
2 teaspoons cider vinegar
1/4 teaspoon hot pepper sauce
Salt and freshly ground pepper to taste
1/2 pound small pasta shells
1 large red bell pepper, thinly sliced
1 large green bell pepper, thinly sliced
3 scallions, white and tender greens, cut into 1/4-inch slices
1 stalk celery, thinly sliced
6 ounces cooked seafood (crabmeat, lobster, shrimp, scallops, or combination)
8 pearl or tiny cherry tomatoes

1. In a screw-top jar combine broth, oil, vinegar, hot pepper sauce, and salt and pepper. Close jar tightly and shake until thoroughly combined. Set aside.
2. Cook pasta in a large pot full of boiling water (salted, if desired) until al dente. Drain and allow to cool to room temperature.

3. In a large bowl combine all vegetables and pasta and toss. Add seafood and spoon dressing over all. Toss very gently. Garnish with tomatoes and serve.

SERVES 4

Per serving: 310 calories; 17.0 grams protein; 49.5 grams carbohydrates; 4.6 grams fat; 65 milligrams cholesterol; 100 milligrams sodium (without salting).

SOBA NOODLES WITH SHREDDED DAIKON AND ORANGE SEGMENTS

Soba noodles are Japanese buckwheat noodles. They're beige in color and have a chewy texture. I like to prepare them with an orange-flavored dressing and toss them with shreds of daikon radish. Orange segments add an extra fillip of color as well as taste.

1/2 pound soba noodles
2 cups shredded daikon (Asian radish)
2 small seedless oranges, peeled and segmented
1/2 cup orange juice
2 tablespoons seasoned rice wine vinegar
2 teaspoons low sodium soy sauce
1 teaspoon sesame oil
   Freshly ground pepper to taste
1 small cucumber, diced
1 plum tomato, diced

1. In a large pot full of boiling water (salted, if desired) cook soba noodles for about 5 minutes or until al dente. Drain and rinse under cold water.

2. Combine noodles, daikon, and orange sections in a bowl and toss.

3. Combine orange juice, vinegar, soy sauce, sesame oil, and pepper in a small bowl and mix until thoroughly combined. Spoon dressing over noodles and toss again to coat ingredients.

4. Transfer noodle mixture to a platter or individual dishes, garnish with cucumber and tomato, and serve.

SERVES 4

Per serving: 255 calories; 9.0 grams protein; 53.0 grams carbohydrates; 1.6 grams fat; 0 milligrams cholesterol; 560 milligrams sodium (without salting).

RICE NOODLES
WITH FRESH GINGERED TUNA

Broiled cubes of tuna, seasoned with grated ginger, crown a mound of delicate rice noodles dressed in a blend of sesame oil, vinegar, soy sauce, garlic, and sugar for an Asian-oriented salad that is both low in fat and inscrutably delicious. Dig into this salad as a main course at lunch or present it as an addition to a party buffet.

1/2 pound long rice noodles (rice vermicelli)
3/4 pound tuna steak, about 1-inch thick
1/2 tablespoon grated peeled ginger
  Salt and freshly ground pepper to taste
1/2 teaspoon sesame oil
 2 tablespoons white vinegar
 2 teaspoons low sodium soy sauce
 1 clove garlic, pressed
1/2 teaspoon sugar
 2 cups shredded romaine lettuce
 1 tablespoon chopped fresh cilantro

1. Preheat broiler.

2. In a large pot full of boiling water (salt, if desired), cook rice noodles for about 5 minutes or until al dente. Drain, rinsing well under cold water, and transfer to a large bowl.

3. Season tuna steak with ginger and salt and pepper to taste. Place on a broiler pan and broil for

about 5 minutes on each side, or until cooked. Remove from broiler and set aside to cool.

4. While tuna cools, combine sesame oil, vinegar, soy sauce, garlic, and sugar in a jar with a screw top. Close jar tightly and shake until dressing is thoroughly blended.

5. Spoon half the dressing over the rice noodles and toss lightly.

6. Arrange romaine lettuce on a serving platter. Heap rice noodles in the center of the platter.

7. Cube tuna and arrange pieces on top of the vermicelli. Spoon remainder of dressing over fish, garnish with cilantro, and serve.

SERVES 4

Per serving: 315 calories; 23.0 grams protein; 51.0 grams carbohydrates; 1.8 grams fat; 47 milligrams cholesterol; 145 milligrams sodium (without salting).

CURRIED RICE AND CANTALOUPE SALAD WITH YOGURT DRESSING

Any sweet orange-fleshed melon from the musk-melon family can be used for this recipe. The sweetness of the melon will balance the slight heat of the cayenne and curry, adding just the right counterpoint.

  1 cup rice
  2 cups water
  1 cup low fat plain yogurt
  2 teaspoons curry powder or to taste
  1 clove garlic, pressed
  1 tablespoon minced fresh cilantro
  ¼ cup low fat (1%) milk
     Pinch cayenne pepper or to taste
     Salt to taste
  1 cup cubed cantaloupe

1. Combine rice and water in a medium heavy saucepan with a lid. Cover and bring to a boil. Lower heat to a simmer and cook for 15 to 20 minutes or until rice is tender and liquid is absorbed. If rice is not tender and liquid has been absorbed add more water, ¼ cup at a time. Remove rice from heat, fluff with a fork, and allow to return to room temperature.

2. While rice cooks, combine all remaining ingre-

dients, except for cantaloupe, in a small bowl. Mix thoroughly.

3. Add cantaloupe to rice and transfer to a serving bowl. Pour yogurt dressing over rice and mix to combine. Cover and chill before serving.

Serves 4

Per serving: 230 calories; 7.5 grams protein; 46.0 grams carbohydrates; 1.6 grams fat; 4 milligrams cholesterol; 55 milligrams sodium (without salting).

ORANGE-FLAVORED RICE WITH FENNEL AND ARUGULA

The slightly anise flavor of raw fennel is terrific in this bright-tasting salad. Peppery arugula plays well off this combination, providing yet another layer of complexity. If fennel is unavailable, use celery instead.

1 cup rice
2 cups water
3 tablespoons orange juice
1 teaspoon grated orange rind
2 teaspoons olive oil
1 cup thinly sliced fennel
1/2 teaspoon cracked black pepper or to taste
    Salt to taste
1 small bunch arugula, trimmed and separated into
    leaves

1. Combine rice and water in a medium heavy saucepan. Cover and bring to a boil. Lower heat to a simmer and cook 15 to 20 minutes or until rice is tender and liquid is absorbed. Remove rice from heat and set aside to cool to room temperature.

2. Combine orange juice, orange rind, and oil in a large bowl. Add fennel, cracked pepper, and salt to taste and mix until thoroughly combined.

3. Fluff rice with a fork and add to fennel and dressing in bowl, mixing well.

4. Place arugula leaves on a serving platter, spoon rice into the center of the platter, and serve.

SERVES 4

Per serving: 205 calories; 4.0 grams protein; 40.0 grams carbohydrates; 3.2 grams fat; 0 milligrams cholesterol; 25 milligrams sodium (without salting).

SESAME RICE SALAD

To toast sesame seeds, heat a nonstick skillet and pour the sesames in—without oil—cooking them until they turn golden brown. The sesame seeds add yet another layer of crunch and taste to a salad loaded with it. Serve at room temperature or slightly chilled.

3 cups cooked basmati brown rice, at room
    temperature
6 scallions, white and tender greens, sliced
4 ounces fresh snow peas, trimmed and cut in to strips
1 red bell pepper, seeded and cut into thin strips
1 cucumber, preferably Kirby, peeled, seeded, and
    thinly sliced
1/2 cup sliced water chestnuts, fresh or canned and
    drained
2 tablespoons sesame seeds, toasted
1/4 cup Low Fat Chicken Stock (page 3) or canned low
    sodium broth
2 tablespoons rice wine vinegar
2 tablespoons low sodium soy sauce
2 teaspoons sesame oil
1 teaspoon peanut or olive oil
    Salt and freshly ground pepper to taste

1. Combine rice, scallions, snow peas, bell pepper, cucumber, water chestnuts, and sesame seeds in a large bowl. Toss lightly and set aside.
2. Combine all remaining ingredients in a small jar

with a lid or a bowl. Shake jar vigorously or whisk well.

3. Pour dressing over rice and toss lightly to combine ingredients.

SERVES 6

Per serving: 170 calories; 4.0 grams protein; 28.5 grams carbohydrates; 4.5 grams fat; 0 milligrams cholesterol; 215 milligrams sodium (without salting).

BARLEY AND CORN TOSS
IN LETTUCE CUPS

Kernels of corn add a touch of sweetness and texture to this salad that tastes as though it could have been born and bred in the Heartland of America.

This heart-healthy, lovely-looking dish works well as a first course or as a side dish with grilled seafood, meat, or poultry.

1/2 cup barley
1 cup cooked corn kernels, fresh or frozen
1 small onion, minced
  Salt and freshly ground pepper to taste
2 tablespoons seasoned rice wine vinegar
1 tablespoon olive oil
4 large crisp lettuce leaves (iceberg or Bibb)
4 pearl tomatoes or 2 cherry tomatoes cut in half

1. Cook barley in a medium saucepan full of water for 30 to 40 minutes or until tender. Drain in a colander and rinse under cold water. Drain again.

2. Combine barley, corn, and onion in a large bowl. Mix and season to taste with salt and pepper.

3. Combine vinegar and oil in a screw-top jar. Shake until blended and spoon gradually over barley, stirring so that dressing is evenly distributed over ingredients.

4. Refrigerate for at least 1 hour to chill salad.

5. Just before serving place a lettuce leaf on each

salad plate. Spoon barley salad into lettuce and top each serving with a pearl tomato.

SERVES 4
Per serving: 150 calories; 3.5 grams protein; 24.5 grams carbohydrates; 4.3 grams fat; 0 milligrams cholesterol; 10 milligrams sodium (without salting).

COUSCOUS SALAD
WITH ENDIVE AND RAISINS

An herbal balsamic vinaigrette adds spark to this unusual salad, while the raisins, endive, and couscous provide color, flavor, volume, and the vitamins—without the fat!

1¼ cups Low Fat Chicken Stock (page 3) or canned low
    sodium broth
 ¼ cup fresh lemon juice
 1 cup quick-cooking couscous
   Salt and freshly ground pepper to taste
 1 endive, coarsely chopped
 1 tablespoon golden raisins
 2 teaspoons olive oil
 2 teaspoons balsamic vinegar
 1 tablespoon minced fresh mint
 1 tablespoon minced fresh parsley

1. Combine stock and lemon juice in a large saucepan and bring to a boil. Add couscous and salt and pepper, cover, and cook for 2 minutes. Remove from heat and let stand for 5 to 10 minutes or until tender.

2. Combine endive and raisins in a large bowl.

3. Combine oil and vinegar in a screw-top jar and shake until blended. Pour over endive-raisin combination and mix thoroughly.

4. Add couscous to bowl and toss. Add mint and

parsley and toss again. Refrigerate until chilled before serving.

SERVES 4

Per serving: 235 calories; 8.0 grams protein; 43.5 grams carbohydrates; 3.4 grams fat; 2 milligrams cholesterol; 55 milligrams sodium (without salting).

PIZZA

BASIC PIZZA DOUGH

This recipe is for two pizza crusts; even if I need only one crust, I always double the recipe and refrigerate or freeze half after the dough has risen. Zipped in a plastic bag, it can be refrigerated for two days and frozen for up to two months. Bring the dough—frozen or refrigerated—to room temperature before using.

  1 cup warm (105°–110° F.) water
  1 package active dry yeast
2¼ cups unbleached white flour (approximate)
  ½ teaspoon salt
    Olive oil cooking spray

1. Put water in a large warm bowl. Sprinkle with yeast and stir to dissolve. Let stand about 5 minutes. Add 1 cup flour and salt. Mix well. Gradually add a second cup of flour, stirring with a wooden spoon. Continue to add flour by the tablespoonful and mix with hands until dough pulls away from sides of bowl and forms a soft, sticky mass. Remove from bowl and turn out onto a lightly floured surface. Wipe out mixing bowl, coat inner surface with cooking spray, and set aside.

2. Knead dough for 5 minutes or until smooth and no longer sticky, adding small amounts of flour if necessary. Shape dough into ball and return to bowl, rolling it around until coated with a film of oil. Cover bowl and let rise in a warm, draft-free place,

for about 45 minutes or until dough has doubled in bulk.

3. Punch down dough with fist. Peel dough out of bowl and divide into two halves. Knead for 1 minute, return to bowl, and allow dough to rise until doubled again, about 1 hour. Dough is now ready to be shaped, topped, and baked. Or dough can be divided into balls, tightly covered in plastic wrap, and frozen for future use.

MAKES 2 PIZZA CRUSTS (EACH 12- TO 14-INCH DIAMETER)
One crust: 520 calories; 15.0 grams protein; 110.0 grams carbohydrates; 2.5 grams fat; 0 milligrams cholesterol; 535 milligrams sodium (without salting).

HEARTY PIZZA
WITH TURKEY SAUSAGE SAUCE

Fresh tomatoes, nutritious, virtually fat-free, and low in calories, are a great choice for health-conscious foodies. And this tomato-rich sauce contains Italian-style turkey sausage that is relatively low in fat and very high in flavor.

This pizza makes a delightful starter or light lunch; or snack while watching the Big Game on TV.

> Basic Pizza Dough for 1 crust (page 87)
> 1 tablespoon olive oil
> 1 small onion, diced
> 1 clove garlic, pressed
> 6 ounces Italian turkey sausage, casing removed
> 1/2 teaspoon red pepper flakes or to taste
> Salt to taste
> 6 diced ripe plum tomatoes
> Vegetable oil cooking spray
> Cornmeal for pan
> 2 ounces low fat mozzarella cheese, diced

1. Prepare pizza dough through step 3; thaw to room temperature if frozen or refrigerated.

2. Heat oil in a large nonstick skillet. Add onion and garlic and cook, stirring, for 1 minute. Add turkey meat and cook, stirring occasionally, until lightly browned.

3. Add seasonings and tomatoes to skillet. Stir to

combine, cover, and cook over low heat for 30 minutes.

4. Meanwhile, preheat oven to 425° F.

5. Lightly coat a 12- to 14-inch pizza pan with cooking spray and sprinkle with cornmeal. Roll out pizza dough and transfer to pan.

6. Spread meat sauce over pizza. Distribute cheese over sauce.

7. Bake for 15 to 20 minutes or until crust is brown and crisp. Remove from oven and let stand for 1 minute before slicing.

SERVES 4

Per serving: 320 calories; 15.5 grams protein; 37.0 grams carbohydrates; 12.3 grams fat; 50 milligrams cholesterol; 550 milligrams sodium (without salting).

SHRIMP AND MOZZARELLA PIZZA

For those who like tarragon, the herb adds its distinctive aniselike flavor to this shrimp- and cheese-topped pie. If tarragon doesn't appeal to you, substitute parsley, basil, or oregano.

Basic Pizza Dough for 1 crust (page 87)
2 teaspoons olive oil
½ pound shrimp, peeled, deveined, and coarsely chopped
1 clove garlic, pressed
Salt and freshly ground pepper to taste
2 tablespoons no-salt-added tomato paste
1 tablespoon water
¼ teaspoon tarragon or to taste
Vegetable oil cooking spray
Cornmeal for pan
2 ounces low fat mozzarella, diced

1. Prepare pizza dough through step 3; thaw to room temperature if frozen or refrigerated.

2. Heat oil in a large nonstick skillet. Add shrimp and garlic and cook, stirring, over medium-high heat for 3 minutes. Season to taste with salt and pepper and set aside.

3. Preheat oven to 425° F. Lightly coat a 12- to 14-inch pizza pan with cooking spray and sprinkle with cornmeal.

4. Combine tomato paste, water, and tarragon in a small bowl. Mix until thoroughly blended.

5. Roll out pizza dough and transfer to pan.

6. Brush surface of dough with tomato paste mixture. Spread shrimp mixture over pizza and distribute cheese over shrimp.

7. Bake for 15 to 20 minutes or until crust is brown and crisp. Remove from oven and let stand for 1 minute before slicing.

SERVES 4

Per serving: 255 calories; 19.0 grams protein; 30.5 grams carbohydrates; 6.3 grams fat; 92 milligrams cholesterol; 345 milligrams sodium (without salting).

ZUCCHINI AND GRUYÈRE PIZZA

Nothing beats the flavor of the real thing, but if you can't find good fresh Swiss Gruyère, use good domestic Swiss-style cheese.

   Basic Pizza Dough for 1 crust (page 87)
   Vegetable oil cooking spray
   Cornmeal for pan
2 *tablespoons no-salt-added tomato paste*
1 *tablespoon water*
1 *teaspoon minced fresh dill*
2 *ounces Gruyère cheese, shredded*
5 *small zucchini, thinly sliced*
$^1/_2$ *teaspoon freshly ground pepper*
   Salt to taste
2 *teaspoons low fat Parmesan cheese*

1. Prepare pizza dough through step 3; thaw to room temperature if frozen or refrigerated.

2. Preheat oven to 425° F. Coat a 12- to 14-inch pizza pan with cooking spray, sprinkle with cornmeal, and set aside.

3. Combine tomato paste, water, and dill in a small bowl. Mix until thoroughly blended.

4. Roll out pizza dough and transfer to prepared pan.

5. Brush pizza dough with tomato paste mixture. Distribute cheese over pizza.

6. Spread zucchini slices over pizza, season to taste with salt and pepper, and sprinkle with Parmesan.

7. Bake for 15 to 20 minutes or until crust is brown and crisp. Remove from oven and let stand for 1 minute before slicing.

SERVES 4

Per serving: 220 calories; 10.0 grams protein; 32.0 grams carbohydrates; 6.2 grams fat; 16 milligrams cholesterol; 210 milligrams sodium (without salting).

PIZZA WITH DRIED TOMATOES AND FARMER CHEESE

For the uninitiated, farmer cheese is a form of cottage cheese from which most of the liquid has been pressed. Sold in a solid loaf, it has a tangy flavor and is firm enough to slice or crumble and, combined with the scallions, makes a sturdy bed for sun-dried tomatoes.

    Basic Pizza Dough for 1 crust (page 87)
    Vegetable oil cooking spray
    Cornmeal for pan
1 tablespoon olive oil
$\frac{1}{2}$ cup low sodium farmer cheese
3 scallions, white and tender greens, minced
    Salt and freshly ground pepper to taste
2 ounces no-salt-added dried tomatoes (not oil-packed), softened in hot water and diced

1. Prepare pizza dough through step 3; thaw to room temperature if frozen or refrigerated.

2. Preheat oven to 425° F. Lightly coat a 12- to 14-inch pizza pan with cooking spray and sprinkle with cornmeal.

3. Roll out pizza dough and transfer to prepared pan. Brush dough with oil.

4. Combine cheese, scallions, and pepper in a small bowl. Mash together until well mixed.

5. Spread cheese mixture over dough. Distribute tomatoes over cheese.

6. Bake for 15 to 20 minutes or until crust is brown and crisp. Remove from oven and let stand for 1 minute before slicing.

SERVES 4
Per serving: 215 calories; 8.0 grams protein; 30.0 grams carbohydrates; 7.5 grams fat; 10 milligrams cholesterol; 210 milligrams sodium (without salting).

CHICKEN AND RICOTTA PIZZA WITH TOMATOES AND BELL PEPPER

Who would think we could afford to eat a rich and satisfying pizza while watching our arteries, not to mention our waistlines? We can with this one.

Basic Pizza Dough for 1 crust (page 87)
Vegetable oil cooking spray
Cornmeal for pan
1 tablespoon olive oil
1/2 cup shredded cooked chicken breast
1 small bell pepper (green, red, or yellow), chopped
4 plum tomatoes, sliced into rounds
1/4 teaspoon dried thyme
Freshly ground pepper to taste
1/2 cup low fat ricotta cheese

1. Prepare pizza dough through step 3; thaw to room temperature if frozen or refrigerated.
2. Preheat oven to 425° F. Lightly coat a 12- to 14-inch pizza pan with cooking spray and sprinkle with cornmeal.
3. Roll out pizza dough and transfer to a pan. Brush dough with oil.
4. Arrange chicken, bell pepper, and tomato rounds over dough. Season with thyme and salt and pepper and distribute cheese evenly over all.
5. Bake for 15 to 20 minutes or until crust is

brown and crisp. Remove from oven and let stand
for 1 minute before slicing.

SERVES 4

Per serving: 260 calories; 13.0 grams protein; 35.0 grams
carbohydrates; 7.8 grams fat; 20 milligrams cholesterol;
185 milligrams sodium (without salting).

MIXED MUSHROOM PIZZA
WITH GOAT CHEESE

This is a kind of "designer" pizza served in the hot new restaurants of the moment. You can use any combination of wild and domestic mushrooms you desire, but there's just no substitute for the delightfully tart flavor of goat cheese, or *chèvre* as it's called in France.

    Basic Pizza Dough for 1 crust (page 87)
  1 teaspoon olive oil
 ¼ pound white mushrooms, wiped clean and thinly
      sliced
 ¼ pound shiitake mushrooms, wiped clean and thinly
      sliced
  1 clove garlic, pressed
    Salt and freshly ground pepper to taste
    Pinch cayenne pepper, optional
  1 tablespoon finely chopped fresh parsley
    Vegetable oil cooking spray
    Cornmeal for pan
  2 ounces soft goat cheese

1. Prepare pizza dough through step 3; thaw to room temperature if frozen or refrigerated.

2. Heat olive oil in a medium saucepan. Add both mushrooms, garlic, salt and pepper, and cayenne if desired; stir to combine. Cover and cook until mushrooms are just tender and liquid has evaporated. Remove from heat, stir in parsley, and set aside.

3. Preheat oven to 425° F. Lightly coat a 12- to 14-inch pizza pan with cooking spray and sprinkle with cornmeal.

4. Roll out pizza dough and transfer to pan.

5. Spread mushroom mixture evenly over dough. Crumble goat cheese and distribute over pizza.

6. Bake for 15 to 20 minutes or until crust is brown and crisp. Remove from oven and let stand for 1 minute before slicing.

SERVES 4

Per serving: 245 calories; 9.0 grams protein; 39.0 grams carbohydrates; 6.3 grams fat; 10 milligrams cholesterol; 225 milligrams sodium (without salting).

CHEESE-FREE PIZZA WITH CURRIED EGGPLANT AND CILANTRO

This pie will remind you of the savory bread toppings served at fine Indian restaurants. If small Asian or Italian eggplants are unavailable, use the smallest regular ones you can find.

   Basic Pizza Dough for 1 crust (page 87)
   6 small Asian or Italian eggplants (about 1¹/₂ pounds)
   1 tablespoon olive oil
   ¹/₄ cup vegetable broth or stock
   4 plum tomatoes, diced
   1 teaspoon curry powder
   Salt and freshly ground pepper to taste
   Vegetable oil cooking spray
   Cornmeal for pan
   1 tablespoon chopped fresh cilantro

1. Prepare pizza dough through step 3; thaw to room temperature if frozen or refrigerated.

2. Remove stems from eggplants but do not peel. Slice each eggplant horizontally into ¹/₄-inch slices.

3. Heat olive oil in a large nonstick skillet. Add eggplant and sauté over medium heat, turning once, for 3 minutes.

4. Add stock, tomatoes, curry powder, and salt and pepper to skillet. Cover and cook for about 20 minutes or until eggplant is tender.

5. Meanwhile, preheat oven to 425° F. Lightly coat

a 12- to 14-inch pizza pan with cooking spray and sprinkle with cornmeal.

6. Roll out pizza dough and transfer to pan.

7. Spread eggplant-tomato mixture evenly over dough.

8. Bake for 15 to 20 minutes or until crust is brown and crisp. Remove from oven and sprinkle with cilantro. Let stand for 1 minute before slicing.

SERVES 4

Per serving: 235 calories; 6.0 grams protein; 42.0 grams carbohydrates; 5.6 grams fat; 0 milligrams cholesterol; 155 milligrams sodium (without salting).

THE MAIN DISH:
MEAT AND POULTRY

PASTA BOLOGNESE

The classic version of this dish originated in Bologna, a city in northern Italy where the use of fresh ingredients is mandatory, as is the case throughout this food-conscious country. It is here, in the north, that cream and butter are used in abundance. Traditionally, then, this rich, luxurious creation contains butter and oil, pancetta (Italian bacon), lots of meat, and a generous amount of heavy cream. My slimmed-down adaptation is no less tasty, but its flavor relies heavily on fresh vegetables and herbs and only minimally upon the meat. Also, I've omitted the butter and cream and only hinted at the olive oil.

2 teaspoons olive oil
2 carrots, finely diced or shredded
1 celery stalk, finely diced
1 medium onion, finely diced
2 cloves garlic, finely minced
2 tablespoons chopped fresh Italian parsley
1/2 pound ground lean turkey or veal
1/4 cup dry white wine
1/4 cup Low Fat Chicken Stock (page 3) or canned low
    sodium broth
1 can (28 ounces) no-salt-added crushed tomatoes
    Salt and freshly ground pepper to taste
1 tablespoon chopped fresh basil or parsley
1/2 pound fettuccine or tagliatelle

6 fresh basil leaves or 2 tablespoons chopped fresh
 parsley for garnish
1 tablespoon grated low fat Parmesan cheese, optional

1. Heat oil in a large nonstick skillet. Add carrots, celery, and onion, and cook over medium heat, stirring frequently, for 3 minutes.

2. Add garlic, parsley, and turkey or veal. Cook, breaking up and separating meat, for 10 minutes.

3. Add wine, stock, tomatoes with its juice, salt and pepper, and basil to skillet. Stir to combine ingredients. Cover, reduce heat to low, and simmer, stirring occasionally, for about 30 minutes or until nearly all liquid has been absorbed.

4. About 10 minutes before sauce is ready, cook pasta in a large pot full of boiling water (salted, if desired) until al dente. Drain, reserving about 2 tablespoons of cooking liquid. Return pasta to pot, add reserved cooking liquid, and toss.

5. Transfer hot pasta to center of a large serving platter or bowl. Spoon sauce over pasta, garnish with basil or parsley, and sprinkle with Parmesan cheese if desired.

SERVES 4

Per serving: 390 calories; 20.0 grams protein; 58.5 grams carbohydrates; 8.0 grams fat; 43 milligrams cholesterol; 115 milligrams sodium (without salting).

FETTUCCINE AND EGGPLANT WITH CUBED STEAK

You can substitute lean turkey breast for the beef, if you prefer poultry to red meat, or you could eliminate the meat altogether when you're in a vegetarian frame of mind—and either the meat or meatless version would be just as good served over bulgur or polenta. However, the eggplants, tomatoes, onion, garlic, and thyme are nonnegotiable items in this marvelous Mediterranean-style dish.

1 tablespoon olive oil
³/₄ pound lean top round steak, fat removed, cut into
    ¹/₂-inch cubes
1 large onion, diced
2 cloves garlic, pressed
2 medium ripe tomatoes, diced
4 small Asian eggplants (about 1 pound total)
¹/₂ teaspoon dried thyme
    Salt and freshly ground pepper to taste
¹/₂ cup canned low sodium beef broth or consomme
³/₄ pound fettuccine

1. Heat oil in a large nonstick skillet. Add beef and brown on all sides over medium-high heat for about 5 minutes. Using a slotted spoon remove beef from skillet and set aside to drain on paper towels.

2. Add onion, garlic, and tomatoes to skillet. Cook over low heat, stirring occasionally, for 5 minutes.

3. Remove stems from eggplant and cube; do not

peel. (These small eggplant have so mild a flavor that they don't have to be peeled or seeded.) Add eggplant, thyme, and salt and pepper to skillet. Cover and cook over low heat for 5 minutes.

4. Add beef cubes and stock to skillet. Cover and let simmer, stirring occasionally, for about 30 minutes or until beef is tender and ingredients are blended. If too much liquid evaporates, add additional broth or a little water to skillet.

5. While sauce simmers, cook fettuccine in a large pot full of boiling water (salted, if desired) until al dente. Drain.

6. Add fettuccine to skillet and stir to combine with sauce. Taste and correct seasoning, if necessary, and serve directly from the skillet or transfer to a heated platter.

SERVES 6
Per serving: 340 calories; 16.5 grams protein; 51.5 grams carbohydrates; 7.4 grams fat; 24 milligrams cholesterol; 40 milligrams sodium (without salting).

ZITI WITH VEAL
AND VEGETABLE PUREE

This is a slimmed-down version of the very rich Genovese-style sauce that is made with oil and butter, carrots, celery, veal, wine and heavy cream. By pureeing the vegetables, you get the sense of richness without the fat (and, as a bonus, the cooking time is cut by about 75 percent).

Rigatoni, penne, or mostaccioli may be substituted for the ziti.

   2 medium carrots, cut into 1-inch pieces
   2 small zucchini, cut into 2-inch pieces
   2 stalks celery, cut into 2-inch pieces
   $^1/_2$ cup Low Fat Chicken Stock (page 3) or canned low
        sodium broth
   $^1/_4$ teaspoon dried oregano
   2 teaspoons olive oil
   $^1/_2$ pound ground veal
   $^1/_4$ teaspoon hot pepper flakes (or to taste)
        Salt and freshly ground pepper to taste
   $^1/_2$ pound ziti

1. Combine vegetables, stock, and oregano in a food processor. Process until coarsely pureed and set aside.

2. Heat oil in a large nonstick skillet. Add veal and sauté over medium-high heat, stirring, for about 5 minutes or until meat no longer looks raw.

3. Add vegetable puree to veal in skillet and stir to

combine. Add hot pepper flakes and salt and pepper to taste. Cover, reduce heat to low, and let simmer for 15 minutes.

4. While sauce simmers, cook ziti in a large pot full of boiling water (salted, if desired) until al dente.

5. Drain pasta and place in a large bowl. Spoon sauce over pasta gradually, tossing to combine. Taste and correct seasoning if necessary before serving.

SERVES 4

Per serving: 340 calories; 19.5 grams protein; 48.0 grams carbohydrates; 7.5 grams fat; 47 milligrams cholesterol; 90 milligrams sodium (without salting).

LASAGNA WITH LEEKS, MUSHROOMS, AND SCALLOPINE OF VEAL

Here's a cheese-free lasagna with lots of character. If you miss the cheese, add a sprinkling of grated low fat Parmesan or Romano before putting the lasagna in the oven, or pass the cheese and those who wish it can add some.

1 tablespoon olive oil
1 tablespoon mild paprika or to taste
1 pound veal scallopine, cut into thin strips
2 leeks, white and tender greens, chopped
3/4 pound mushrooms, wiped clean and thinly sliced
2 cloves garlic, minced
1 tablespoon fresh lemon juice
1 1/2 cups canned low sodium beef broth
3/4 cup canned no-salt-added tomato sauce
1/4 teaspoon hot pepper flakes or to taste
1 tablespoon chopped fresh parsley
Salt to taste
3/4 pound lasagna noodles

1. Preheat oven to 350° F.
2. Heat oil in a large nonstick skillet. Sprinkle paprika on veal strips and add to skillet. Sauté over medium-high heat, stirring constantly, for about 3 minutes or until veal is cooked through. Remove veal from skillet with a slotted spoon and set aside.
3. Add leeks, mushrooms, and garlic to skillet.

Sprinkle with lemon juice and sauté, stirring, for 3 minutes.

4. Add stock, tomato sauce, pepper flakes, parsley, and salt to skillet. Cover, reduce heat to medium-low and cook for about 5 minutes or until mushrooms are just tender. Remove from heat, correct seasonings if necessary, and set aside.

5. In a large pot full of boiling water cook pasta until just al dente. (Pasta will be baked, so don't overcook.) Drain.

6. Assemble dish in a nonstick baking dish or casserole. Start with a spoonful of sauce and create layers of lasagna, veal, and mushrooms. Repeat until all ingredients have been used. The final layer should be lasagna. Cover with foil and bake for about 20 minutes or until ingredients are heated through. Serve hot from the baking pan.

SERVES 6

Per serving: 370 calories; 26.0 grams protein; 53.5 grams carbohydrates; 5.7 grams fat; 60 milligrams cholesterol; 90 milligrams sodium (without salting).

LINGUINE WITH ASPARAGUS AND PROSCIUTTO

I favor using shallots over onions here for their mild onion flavor. Fresh "green" shallots are available in the spring, but as is true with garlic and onions, dry shallots (that is, with dry skins and moist flesh) are available throughout the year. Fresh shallots can be refrigerated for up to a week, while dry shallots may be stored in a cool, dry place for up to a month.

Regular or spinach linguine would work fine here, but if whole wheat linguine is available, please try it—it complements the flavors in this dish beautifully.

1/2 pound linguine, preferably whole wheat
2 teaspoons olive oil
8 large asparagus, tough stalks removed, cut in half lengthwise and then into 2-inch lengths
2 shallots, minced
1 clove garlic, pressed
6 plum tomatoes, diced
1 cup Low Fat Chicken Stock (page 3) or canned low sodium broth
2 ounces lean prosciutto, thinly sliced and cut into narrow strips
Salt and freshly ground pepper to taste
1 tablespoon grated low fat Parmesan cheese, optional

1. Put pasta up to cook in a large pot full of boiling water (salted, if desired) until al dente.

2. While pasta cooks, heat oil in a large nonstick skillet. Add asparagus and shallots and sauté over medium-high heat, stirring, for 2 minutes. Add garlic, tomatoes, and stock and bring to a boil. Reduce heat to medium and simmer for 5 minutes.

3. Stir prosciutto into skillet and cook an additional minute to heat through. Season to taste with salt and pepper.

4. Drain linguine and transfer into a large serving bowl. Spoon sauce over pasta and toss to combine. Sprinkle with grated cheese, if desired, and serve immediately.

SERVES 4

Per serving: 325 calories; 13.0 grams protein; 51.5 grams carbohydrates; 7.7 grams fat; 9 milligrams cholesterol; 290 milligrams sodium (without salting).

ANGEL HAIR PASTA
AND CHICKEN BAKED
IN YOGURT

The rich taste belies the stingy fat-count in this creamy, though not creamed, baked dish. The flour will keep the yogurt from breaking down while cooking, so it's a very important ingredient to remember.

2 teaspoons olive oil
1 pound skinless and boneless chicken breasts, cubed
$^1/_4$ pound mushrooms, wiped clean and thinly sliced
$^1/_2$ cup dry white wine
2 tablespoons chopped flat-leaf (Italian) parsley
  Salt and freshly ground pepper to taste
$^3/_4$ pound angel hair pasta or cappellini
$^1/_2$ cup low fat (1%) milk
$^1/_2$ cup low fat plain yogurt
2 teaspoons all-purpose flour
1 tablespoon grated low fat Parmesan cheese

1. Preheat oven to 350° F.
2. Heat oil in a large nonstick skillet. Add chicken cubes and brown on all sides over medium-high heat for about 5 minutes. Add mushrooms, wine, parsley, and salt and pepper and bring to a boil. Cover, reduce heat to low and simmer, stirring occasionally, for about 7 minutes or until chicken is done and mushrooms are tender.
3. While chicken simmers, cook pasta in a large

pot full of boiling water (salted, if desired) until al dente. Drain and place in a large bowl.

4. In a small bowl combine milk, yogurt, and flour. Mix until thoroughly combined.

5. Add chicken mixture from skillet to pasta and toss.

6. Spoon milk-yogurt combination over all ingredients and toss again. Taste and correct seasoning if necessary.

7. Spoon pasta-chicken mixture into a baking dish or ovenproof casserole and sprinkle with grated cheese. Cover and bake for 20 minutes. Remove cover and bake an additional 5 minutes. Serve immediately.

SERVES 6
Per serving: 340 calories; 28.0 grams protein; 46.0 grams carbohydrates; 4.3 grams fat; 45 milligrams cholesterol; 100 milligrams sodium (without salting).

GINGERED NOODLES
WITH CHICKEN

Chinese noodle shop aficionados will be reminded of Cantonese Noodles (wide, flat, soft rice noodles) with Chicken. This adaptation is ideal for low fat schemes since you control the amount of oil used.

$^1/_2$ pound skinless and boneless chicken breasts,
    shredded
1 large onion, cut in half lengthwise and thinly sliced
1 stalk celery, sliced
1 carrot, diced
3 cups Low Fat Chicken Stock (page 3) or canned low
    sodium broth
$1^1/_2$ tablespoons low sodium soy sauce
1 teaspoon sesame oil
1 tablespoon grated peeled ginger root
    Salt and freshly ground pepper to taste
$^1/_2$ pound broad noodles
1 tablespoon cornstarch
$^1/_4$ cup cold water
2 tablespoons minced fresh parsley

1. Combine all ingredients, except noodles, cornstarch, water, and parsley in a large soup pot and bring to a boil. Cover, reduce heat to low, and simmer gently, stirring occasionally, for 15 minutes.

2. Add noodles to pot and return to a boil. Reduce heat to medium and simmer, uncovered, for about 8 minutes or until noodles are tender.

3. Dissolve cornstarch in cold water and stir into pot. Simmer, stirring, for 1 or 2 minutes or until sauce thickens. Serve in heated bowls garnished with parsley.

SERVES 4

Per serving: 350 calories; 23.0 grams protein; 52.0 grams carbohydrates; 5.5 grams fat; 90 milligrams cholesterol; 340 milligrams sodium (without salting).

CHICKEN MEE FUN

In Chinese "fun" means "noodles." And just about everybody seems to enjoy Chinese noodles these days—which is lots of fun indeed. *Mee fun*, thin rice noodles, are the heart of this full-flavored dish that features the wonderful soul of Chinese cooking. Dried black mushrooms are softened, slivered, and stir-fried with chicken, crisp and crinkly Napa cabbage, and scallions. Use spaghettini, angel hair, or other narrow pasta if rice noodles are unavailable.

  1 ounce dried shiitake or black Chinese mushrooms
  2 teaspoons vegetable or olive oil
    Salt to taste
  4 scallions, white and tender greens, cut diagonally
      into 1-inch pieces
 1/2 pound cooked boneless chicken breasts, fat removed,
      cut into 1-inch strips
  1 small head Napa or savoy cabbage (about 1 pound),
      cut crosswise into 1-inch pieces
 3/4 pound Chinese rice noodles (mee fun) or thin
      spaghetti, parboiled and drained
  1 tablespoon low sodium soy or tamari sauce
  4 tablespoons Low Fat Chicken Stock (page 3) or
      canned low sodium broth (approximate)

1. Soak mushrooms in warm water for 20 minutes. Drain, rinse, and squeeze dry. Remove stems, slice thin, and set aside.

2. Heat oil in a large, heavy nonstick skillet or wok

until very hot. Add salt to taste and scallions and stir-fry for about 30 seconds. Add chicken and stir-fry for an additional 30 to 45 seconds.

3. Add cabbage and reserved mushrooms to skillet or wok and cook for 2 minutes, scooping and tossing gently to thoroughly combine ingredients.

4. Add the cooked noodles, soy or tamari sauce, and 1 tablespoon stock and cook for 1 minute, separating noodles and tossing gently.

5. Cover and reduce heat to medium-low. Cook, stirring frequently and adding additional stock by the tablespoonful if too dry, for about 5 minutes or until ingredients are combined and heated through.

6. Transfer to a heated platter and serve.

SERVES 6

Per serving: 290 calories; 10.5 grams protein; 58.0 grams carbohydrates; 2.0 grams fat; 22 milligrams cholesterol; 150 milligrams sodium (without salting).

WHOLE WHEAT PASTA WITH SMOKED TURKEY AND FENNEL

Celery or celeriac makes a fine substitute for the fennel. If you make that switch, use celery seeds, but do so sparingly.

2 teaspoons olive oil
1 small fennel bulb, trimmed and thinly sliced
1/4 pound skinless smoked turkey breast, diced
1/4 teaspoon crushed fennel seeds
4 scallions, with tops, chopped
1 cup Low Fat Chicken Stock (page 3) or canned low sodium broth
1/2 pound whole wheat pasta (any shape)
Salt and freshly ground pepper to taste

1. Heat oil in a large nonstick skillet. Add fennel and turkey breast to skillet, and sauté over medium-high heat, stirring, for 3 minutes.

2. Add fennel seeds, scallions, and stock to skillet. Cover, reduce heat to low and simmer for 3 minutes. Remove from heat and set aside.

3. Cook pasta in a large pot full of boiling water (salted, if desired) until al dente. Drain.

4. Add pasta to skillet and toss to combine with turkey and fennel. Season to taste with salt and pepper and heat through before serving.

Per serving: 285 calories; 14.0 grams protein; 46.5 grams carbohydrates; 4.0 grams fat; 12 milligrams cholesterol; 345 milligrams sodium (without salting).

BAKED RICE AND LAMB WITH TOMATOES AND HOT PEPPER

Meat from the leg of lamb is one of the leanest you can buy and adds its distinctive taste to the somewhat spicy, full-flavored dish.

2 teaspoons olive oil
• ³/₄ pound lean lamb, preferably from leg, cut into
    ¹/₂-inch cubes
  Salt and freshly ground pepper to taste
1 cup rice
2 ripe tomatoes, cut into wedges
1 small hot cherry pepper, seeded and diced
2 cups Low Fat Chicken Stock (page 3) or canned low
    sodium broth
2 tablespoons chopped fresh basil or parsley

1. Preheat oven to 350° F.
2. Heat oil in a large nonstick skillet. Add lamb and brown lightly on all sides over high heat. Using a slotted spoon transfer lamb to a baking dish or ovenproof casserole and season with salt and pepper.
3. Add rice to lamb and distribute tomato and hot pepper pieces over rice. Pour stock over rice and lamb. Cover and bake for 30 to 40 minutes or until lamb and rice are tender and the liquid has been absorbed. If liquid is absorbed before lamb and rice are cooked add 2 to 3 tablespoons of water or stock.
4. Sprinkle with basil or parsley and serve hot.

SERVES 4

Per serving: 340 calories; 22.5 grams protein; 44.0 grams carbohydrates; 7.9 grams fat; 60 milligrams cholesterol; 205 milligrams sodium (without salting).

LEMONY RICE AND CHICKEN

Rice and chicken is a combination known to nearly every ethnic group in the world. Only the seasonings and cooking techniques may change. But the results are always delicious and treasured. This rice and chicken dish was inspired by many different cuisines, including those of Greece, China, Spain, and France.

I like to serve this multicultural, complexly flavored main course with a salad of bitter greens dressed with balsamic vinaigrette.

2 teaspoons olive oil
1/2 pound skinless and boneless chicken breast, thinly sliced
    Salt and freshly ground pepper to taste
1 stalk celery, thinly sliced
2 cloves garlic, pressed
1 cup rice
2 cups Low Fat Chicken Stock (page 3) or canned low sodium broth
1 teaspoon fresh lemon juice
1/4 teaspoon thyme
1 large lemon, thinly sliced

1. Heat oil in a large nonstick skillet. Add chicken slices and sauté until chicken is white. Remove chicken with a slotted spoon, season to taste with salt and pepper, and set aside.

2. Add celery, garlic, and rice to skillet. Cook, stirring over medium heat, for 2 minutes.

3. Return chicken to skillet. Add stock, lemon juice, and thyme. Cover, reduce heat and simmer for about 15 minutes or until liquid is almost completely absorbed and rice is almost cooked.

4. Add lemon slices to skillet, cover and cook an additional 5 minutes or until rice is completely cooked (add additional stock or water if necessary). Season to taste and serve.

SERVES 4
Per serving: 275 calories; 17.0 grams protein; 42.0 grams carbohydrates; 4.1 grams fat; 35 milligrams cholesterol; 80 milligrams sodium (without salting).

BOMBAY RICE AND CHICKEN WITH GREEN BEANS

By combining cardamom, cumin, and turmeric you'll be creating your own homemade curry. Like it spicier? Add some cayenne. Want it sweeter? Try cinnamon. Curry is a wonderful way to add flavor without adding fat—so go to it, and enjoy.

2 teaspoons olive oil
1 2¹/₂-pound chicken, skin and fat removed, cut into 8 pieces
  Salt and freshly ground pepper to taste
1 cup brown rice
1 clove garlic, pressed
¹/₂ teaspoon each: ground cardamom, cumin, and turmeric or to taste
3 cups Low Fat Chicken Stock (page 3) or canned low sodium broth
¹/₂ pound green beans

1. Preheat oven to 350° F.

2. Heat oil in a large ovenproof casserole. Add chicken, season with salt and pepper, and brown lightly on all sides over medium-high heat for about 5 minutes.

3. Add rice, garlic, cardamom, cumin, and turmeric to casserole and stir briefly to combine rice with spices.

4. Add stock to casserole, cover, and place in oven.

Bake for 30 to 40 minutes, or until rice and chicken are tender and cooked through.

5. While chicken bakes, blanch green beans in boiling water for 10 minutes. Drain and add to casserole for final 10 minutes of baking.

SERVES 6

Per serving: 260 calories; 23.5 grams protein; 28.0 grams carbohydrates; 6.0 grams fat; 67 milligrams cholesterol; 110 milligrams sodium (without salting).

RICE-STUFFED TURKEY ROLLS

This is a slimmed-down version of braciole, one of my favorite Italian dishes. The lean turkey breast is wrapped around a very tasty rice and low fat mozzarella filling—a combination that will please anyone eating lighter. I love it with steamed zucchini or lightly sautéed spinach or escarole.

    4 turkey cutlets (about ¾ pound)
      Salt and freshly ground pepper to taste
    ¾ cup cooked brown rice
    2 plum tomatoes, seeded and finely minced
    ¼ cup shredded low fat mozzarella cheese (about 1
       ounce)
    1 tablespoon chopped fresh basil or parsley
    2 teaspoons olive or vegetable oil
      Vegetable oil cooking spray

1. Preheat oven to 350° F.
2. Pound turkey cutlets to a thickness of ¼ inch, season to taste with salt and pepper, and set aside.
3. In a medium bowl, combine rice with tomatoes, cheese, basil, and additional seasoning if desired. Mix well.
4. Spoon equal amounts of rice mixture onto turkey cutlets. Fold sides and roll cutlets, secure seam with toothpicks. Wipe cutlets dry.
5. Heat oil in a large nonstick skillet. Add turkey rolls and cook over high heat for about 5 minutes, turning rolls, until all sides are lightly browned.

6. Transfer turkey rolls to a shallow baking pan coated with cooking spray. Bake for 10 minutes or until turkey is cooked through. Serve immediately.

SERVES 4

Per serving: 205 calories; 24.5 grams protein; 15.5 grams carbohydrates; 5.2 grams fat; 56 milligrams cholesterol; 110 milligrams sodium (without salting).

POLENTA AND HUNTER'S CHICKEN

Here's a quickie variation of that retro favorite, chicken cacciatore. It's equally good with turkey served over pasta or rice.

1½ cups Low Fat Chicken Stock (page 3) or canned low
        sodium broth
  ½ cup yellow cornmeal
  2 teaspoons olive oil
  1 small onion, thinly sliced
  1 skinless and boneless chicken breast (about 1
        pound), cut into 4 pieces
  ½ teaspoon dried oregano
  ½ teaspoon dried marjoram
    Salt and freshly ground pepper to taste
  ¼ cup dry red wine
  2 ripe tomatoes, chopped

1. To make polenta, heat stock in a medium sauce-pan and bring to a boil. Stir in cornmeal gradually, and cook, stirring frequently, for about 10 to 20 minutes or until polenta thickens and pulls away from sides of saucepan. Spoon polenta into a shallow pan and set aside to cool slightly.

2. While polenta cooks, heat oil in a large nonstick skillet. Add onion and cook over medium heat, stirring, for 2 minutes. Add chicken, oregano, marjoram, salt and pepper, and wine. Cook, turning chicken once or twice, until wine is reduced by half.

3. Add tomatoes to skillet. Cover, reduce heat, and simmer over low heat until chicken is tender and tomatoes have combined with pan juices, about 15 minutes. Taste and correct seasoning if necessary.

4. Cut polenta into squares and place on 4 dinner plates. Spoon chicken and sauce over and around polenta and serve.

SERVES 4

Per serving: 225 calories; 28.5 grams protein; 16.5 grams carbohydrates; 5.0 grams fat; 67 milligrams cholesterol; 295 milligrams sodium (without salting).

THE MAIN DISH:
FISH AND SEAFOOD

ROTELLE AND GRAY SOLE IN LEMON-PARSLEY SAUCE

Did you know there are no commercially harvested sole in United States waters? It's true! Flatfish from U.S. waters marketed as sole is flounder. However, gray sole—which is a major East Coast flounder—*is* a lean and delicate fish that will accommodate the lemon-parsley sauce with grace and aplomb. If you are unable to find gray sole, substitute other flounder or sole.

1 pound fillet of gray sole
    Salt and freshly ground pepper
2 teaspoons all-purpose flour
2 teaspoons olive oil
2 cups Low Fat Chicken Stock (page 3) or canned low
    sodium broth
    Juice of 1/2 lemon
1/4 cup coarsely chopped fresh parsley
1/2 teaspoon dried dill weed
3/4 pound rotelle pasta

1. Season fish fillets with salt and pepper and coat lightly with flour.

2. Heat oil in a large nonstick skillet. Sauté fish until lightly browned on both sides and cooked through. Using a slotted spatula transfer fish from skillet to paper towel and set aside.

3. Add stock, lemon juice, parsley, and dill to skil-

let. Bring to a simmer and cook, stirring frequently, for 2 minutes.

4. While sauce simmers, cook pasta in a large pot full of boiling water (salted, if desired) until al dente. Drain and add to skillet. Toss to combine ingredients.

5. Place fish fillet on top of pasta in skillet. Cover skillet and heat all ingredients through.

6. Carefully arrange fish fillets around perimeter of a heated serving platter. Spoon pasta and sauce into center of platter and serve.

SERVES 4
Per serving: 295 calories; 27.5 grams protein; 33.5 grams carbohydrates; 5.2 grams fat; 57 milligrams cholesterol; 130 milligrams sodium (without salting).

SPAGHETTINI AND SALMON FILLET IN FRESH BASIL SAUCE

This dish is elegant, simple, and pristine. Here, the play of textures and colors in the fish, pasta, and sauce is wonderful. You may substitute just about any thin pasta for the spaghettini. You must have the salmon, though, for it adds flair as well as flavor.

2 teaspoons olive oil
2 cloves garlic, pressed
1 small carrot, finely diced
   Salt and freshly ground black pepper to taste
2 cups Low Fat Chicken Stock (page 3) or canned low
   sodium broth
2 teaspoons balsamic vinegar
1/2 cup chopped fresh basil leaves
1 pound salmon fillet, cut into 4 pieces
2 tablespoons chopped fresh dill
1/2 teaspoon whole peppercorns
1/2 pound spaghettini

1. Heat oil in a large nonstick skillet. Add garlic, carrot, and salt and pepper. Cook over low heat, stirring, for 2 minutes. Add stock, vinegar, and half of the basil to skillet. Cover and cook over low heat for 15 to 20 minutes, or until sauce is reduced by about one-third.

2. When sauce is almost ready, cook spaghettini in

a large pot full of boiling water (salted, if desired) until al dente.

3. While pasta cooks, place fish in a shallow saucepan or skillet with water to cover. Add dill and peppercorns and bring water to a boil. Reduce heat to a simmer and cook for about 5 minutes, or until fish is cooked through.

4. Drain pasta and place in a large bowl. Spoon half the sauce over the pasta and toss to combine. Transfer pasta to the center of a large heated serving platter.

5. Using a slotted spatula, transfer salmon to platter, arranging pieces beside pasta. Spoon remaining sauce over fish, garnish with remaining basil, and serve immediately.

SERVES 4

Per serving: 410 calories; 30.5 grams protein; 45.5 grams carbohydrates; 11.5 grams fat; 65 milligrams cholesterol; 100 milligrams sodium (without salting).

FETTUCCINE AND SHRIMP WITH STEAMED ARUGULA

Don't be afraid to experiment or make like substitutions in recipes. For example, I've enjoyed this dish using sea scallops instead of shrimp, and escarole, watercress, or spinach leaves for the arugula. The secret is to use quality ingredients whose taste you are familiar with and, of course, enjoy eating.

    1 small bunch arugula, trimmed
    2 teaspoons olive oil
    4 shallots, minced
    6 plum tomatoes, chopped
    1/4 cup dry white wine
    1/2 cup low sodium vegetable or chicken stock or broth
    1/2 pound medium shrimp, shelled, deveined, and cut in
        half lengthwise
    1/2 pound fettuccine
    Salt and freshly ground pepper to taste

1. Separate arugula leaves and rinse thoroughly. Do not drain.

2. Place arugula leaves in a large nonstick skillet. Cover and cook over medium-high heat for 1 minute or until leaves are just wilted. Remove arugula from skillet with a slotted spatula and set aside to drain on paper towels.

3. Dry skillet and heat oil. Add shallots and sauté, stirring, for 1 minute.

4. Add tomatoes, wine, and stock to skillet and bring to a boil. Reduce heat to medium-low, cover, and simmer for 5 minutes.

5. Meanwhile, cook fettuccine in a large pot full of boiling water (salted, if desired) until al dente.

6. Add shrimp to skillet and cook, stirring, for 3 to 4 minutes or until shrimp is cooked through. Remove skillet from heat and set aside.

7. Drain fettuccine and add to skillet. Add arugula and salt and pepper to skillet. Toss to combine and heat through before serving.

SERVES 4

Per serving: 325 calories; 20.0 grams protein; 50.0 grams carbohydrates; 5.0 grams fat; 87 milligrams cholesterol; 110 milligrams sodium (without salting).

SMALL SHELLS WITH CRABMEAT AND CELERY

Here's a wonderfully refreshing recipe in which celery and tarragon highlight the nutty sweetness of crabmeat. Dungeness crab would be divine if obtainable; if not, substitute lump blue crabmeat in this recipe. But don't use bland, rubbery surimi ("imitation crabmeat"), it just won't make it.

Vegetable oil cooking spray
3 cups coarsely chopped celery
$1/2$ teaspoon dried tarragon or to taste
Salt and freshly ground pepper
$1/4$ cup Low Fat Chicken Stock (page 3) or canned low
    sodium broth
$1/2$ pound small pasta shells
6 ounces crabmeat, cartilage removed, shredded
$1/2$ cup fresh or frozen and thawed tiny green peas
1 tablespoon chopped fresh parsley

1. Coat a large nonstick skillet with cooking spray. Add celery, tarragon, salt and pepper and cook over low heat, stirring, for 1 minute. Add stock, cover, and cook about 15 minutes or until celery is crisp-tender.

2. Cook pasta shells in a medium pot full of boiling water (salted, if desired) until al dente.

3. While pasta cooks, add crabmeat and peas to celery in skillet. Stir, cover, and cook for 5 minutes.

4. Drain pasta and transfer to a large heated serv-

ing bowl. Add celery-crabmeat mixture and toss to combine. Garnish with parsley and serve.

SERVES 4

Per serving: 280 calories; 16.5 grams protein; 47.5 grams carbohydrates; 2.5 grams fat; 26 milligrams cholesterol; 215 milligrams sodium (without salting).

PASTA WITH
SCALLOPS AND KALE

Tastes good, looks good, is good, and contains all the ingredients to make it a dinner-party favorite. Serve it with a small salad, crusty bread, and your favorite wine.

    2 teaspoons olive oil
    3 large shallots, thickly sliced
    1 stalk celery, chopped
    1 small red bell pepper, trimmed, seeded, and cut into
        thin 1-inch strips
    2 cloves garlic, finely minced
    1/2 cup Low Fat Chicken Stock (page 3) or canned low
        sodium broth
    1/4 cup dry white wine
    1/2 pound kale, rinsed, trimmed, and chopped
    1/2 pound sturdy pasta (medium shells, penne, ziti,
        spirals, etc.)
    1/2 pound bay scallops (or sea scallops, quartered),
        rinsed
        Salt and freshly ground pepper to taste

1. Heat oil in a large nonstick skillet. Add shallots, celery, and red pepper and cook, stirring frequently, over medium-high heat for about 5 minutes or until shallots are golden. Add garlic and cook, stirring, for an additional minute.

2. Add broth and wine to skillet and bring to a boil. Reduce heat slightly, add kale and cook, uncov-

ered, stirring frequently, for 5 to 8 minutes or until kale starts to wilt.

3. While vegetables cook, cook pasta in a large pot full of water (salted, if desired) until al dente.

4. Add scallops and salt and pepper to skillet and cook, stirring frequently, for 4 to 5 minutes or until scallops are cooked through. Reduce heat to low.

5. When pasta is cooked, drain and add to skillet. Toss gently to blend ingredients and serve immediately.

SERVES 4

Per serving: 315 calories; 18.5 grams protein; 50.5 grams carbohydrates; 4.3 grams fat; 20 milligrams cholesterol; 130 milligrams sodium (without salting).

MUSSELS OREGANO
OVER WHOLE WHEAT PASTA

For me, the sauce—combining fish stock and wine and the gorgeous liquor from the mussels, garlic, tomatoes, and oregano (Greek for "joy of the mountain")—is nectar for the gods; an elixir from which I never want to be weaned.

Try this great pasta and mussel dish with a big green salad, plenty of fresh bread, and dry sparkling wine or soda water.

Note: Do not scrub and beard the mussels until right before you plan to use them or they will spoil.

    2 dozen mussels, scrubbed and debearded
    1 cup fish stock or clam juice
    1/2 cup water
    2 teaspoons olive oil
    1 clove garlic, pressed
    4 ripe tomatoes, cubed
    1/2 cup dry white wine
    1/4 teaspoon red pepper flakes, optional
    1 tablespoon crushed fresh oregano or 2 teaspoons
        dried
    Salt and freshly ground pepper to taste
    1/2 pound whole wheat pasta (any shape)
    1 lemon, cut into 8 wedges

1. Combine mussels, stock or clam juice, and water in a large saucepan and bring to a slow boil.

Cover and cook for about 5 minutes or until shells have opened. Using a slotted spoon, remove mussels from pot, discarding any that have not opened, and set aside. Strain cooking liquid from mussels into a bowl and set aside.

2. Heat oil in a large skillet. Add garlic and cook over medium heat, stirring, for 1 minute. Add tomatoes, wine, red pepper flakes, oregano, salt and pepper, and reserved cooking liquid. Bring to a boil, then reduce heat to medium, cover and simmer for 15 minutes, or until sauce is reduced slightly and thickened.

3. While sauce simmers, cook pasta in a large pot full of boiling water (salted, if desired) until al dente. Drain and transfer pasta to a heated serving bowl.

4. When sauce is almost ready, stir in reserved mussels and cook briefly to heat through. Spoon sauce with mussels over pasta. Toss to combine and serve hot garnished with lemon wedges.

SERVES 4

Per serving: 300 calories; 13.0 grams protein; 51.0 grams carbohydrates; 4.7 grams fat; 10 milligrams cholesterol; 140 milligrams sodium (without salting).

PENNE WITH CLAMS, GARLIC, AND FRESH TOMATOES

An adage I find useful is: Never overlook the obvious. And nothing is more obvious (or delicious) than this great classic that combines pasta with clams tossed in a very light and aromatic tomato sauce. Low in calories and fat, it makes a terrific main course for even the biggest clam fan in your crowd. Serve with crusty bread for sopping up any sauce that collects in the bottom of the plates.

³/₄ cup dry white wine
³/₄ cup fish stock or clam juice
2 cloves garlic, minced
18 cherrystone or littleneck clams, thoroughly scrubbed
¹/₂ pound penne
6 ripe plum tomatoes, diced, with juices
¹/₄ cup chopped fresh Italian parsley
Salt and freshly ground pepper to taste
Grated low fat Parmesan cheese to taste, optional

1. Combine wine, stock or clam juice, and garlic in a large saucepan and bring to a boil. Add clams and reduce heat slightly. Cover and simmer for about 5 minutes, or until clams have opened. Remove clams with a slotted spoon, discarding any that have not opened. Set aside clams to cool.

2. Cook penne in a large pot full of boiling water (salted, if desired) until al dente. Drain and set aside.

3. While pasta cooks, strain cooking liquid from

clams and return to saucepan. Add tomatoes. Cover and simmer for 5 minutes.

4. Remove clams from shells and add to sauce. Continue to cook, uncovered, for an additional 2 or 3 minutes or until pasta is done.

5. Drain pasta and transfer to a heated serving bowl. Top pasta with clams and sauce and toss to combine. Season to taste before serving. Pass grated cheese, if desired.

SERVES 4
Per serving: 310 calories; 20.0 grams protein; 51.5 grams carbohydrates; 2.5 grams fat; 30 milligrams cholesterol; 80 milligrams sodium (without salting).

SHRIMP LO MEIN

Chinese noodle dishes are served as one-dish meals for lunch or light supper. However, they often appear as one of the courses in an elegant banquet. This tasty lo mein can be prepared in advance and reheated. Chicken may be substituted for the shrimp.

    6 ounces dried lo mein noodles or ½ pound linguine
    2 teaspoons vegetable or olive oil
1½ cups bean sprouts
    1 cup shredded Napa cabbage or bok choy
    ½ pound small shrimp, shelled and deveined
    1 cup shredded scallions
    ½ tablespoon dry sherry or sake
    ½ cup Low Fat Chicken Stock (page 3) or canned low
        sodium broth
    1 tablespoon Asian oyster sauce
    1 tablespoon low sodium soy sauce
    ½ teaspoon sugar
        Freshly ground pepper to taste

1. Cook noodles in a large pot full of boiling water (salt, if desired) or according to package directions until al dente. Drain and set aside.

2. Heat 1 teaspoon oil in a wok or skillet. Add bean sprouts and cabbage and cook, stirring, over medium heat for 1 minute. Remove from wok and transfer to a plate.

3. Heat remaining oil in same wok or skillet. Add

shrimp and scallions. Stir and cook over medium heat until shrimp start to turn pink.

4. Add wine, stock, oyster sauce, soy sauce, sugar, and reserved noodles, bean sprouts, and cabbage to wok or skillet. Toss over medium heat to combine ingredients. Sprinkle with pepper and serve hot.

SERVES 4

Per serving: 335 calories; 21.5 grams protein; 50.0 grams carbohydrates; 5.2 grams fat; 87 milligrams cholesterol; 415 milligrams sodium (without salting).

CASSEROLE OF BROWN RICE
AND COD

This delectable recipe has flavors that remind me of the Middle East, Mediterranean, and Asia—all rolled into a whole world meal. So I may accompany it with an arugula salad dressed with a simple balsamic vinaigrette, or a crisp bean sprout salad tossed with rice wine vinegar, or a cool *tzazki:* diced cucumber and yogurt made pungent with garlic and dill.

2 cups water
1 cup brown rice
2 teaspoons olive oil
2 shallots, minced
2 stalks celery, thinly sliced
1 cup Low Fat Chicken Stock (page 3) or canned low
    sodium broth
$1/4$ cup dry vermouth
$1/4$ teaspoon ground cumin
    Salt and freshly ground pepper to taste
    Vegetable oil cooking spray
1 pound cod fillet, cut into 4 pieces

1. In a medium saucepan, bring water to a boil. Add rice and reduce heat to a simmer. Cover and cook for 30 minutes. Liquid should be absorbed but rice will not be tender at this point.

2. Meanwhile, preheat oven to 350° F.

3. Heat oil in a medium nonstick skillet. Add shal-

lots and celery and cook until celery is just tender. Add stock, vermouth, cumin, and salt and pepper to taste. Bring to a simmer and cook for 3 minutes.

4. Leaving room between fillets, arrange cod in a nonstick baking dish or ovenproof casserole lightly coated with cooking spray. Spoon rice between the fillets. Pour contents of skillet over fish and rice and cover baking dish with foil. Bake for about 30 minutes or until rice is tender and fish is cooked through.

SERVES 4

Per serving: 300 calories; 24.5 grams protein; 39.0 grams carbohydrates; 5.0 grams fat; 50 milligrams cholesterol; 100 milligrams sodium (without salting).

SPICED RICE AND LOBSTER

I've made this dish with monkfish fillet ("poor man's lobster") with excellent results, but shrimp, scallops, or crabmeat can also be substituted for the lobster.

2 teaspoons olive oil
1 small red onion, coarsely chopped
1 small red bell pepper, minced
1 cup rice
$1/2$ teaspoon ground cumin
$1/8$ teaspoon ground cinnamon
Salt and freshly ground pepper to taste
$1^{1}/2$ cups Low Fat Chicken Stock (page 3) or low sodium broth
$1/2$ cup dry vermouth or white wine
$1^{1}/2$ cups diced cooked lobster meat
1 tablespoon chopped fresh cilantro or parsley
1 lemon, thinly sliced

1. Heat oil in a large heavy saucepan. Add onion and bell pepper and cook over medium heat, stirring, for 1 minute.

2. Add rice, cumin, cinnamon, and salt and pepper to saucepan. Cook over medium heat, stirring, for an additional minute.

3. Add stock and vermouth to rice, cover, and bring to a boil. Reduce heat to very low and simmer for 12 to 15 minutes or until rice is almost tender and some liquid remains.

4. Add lobster meat to rice and stir lightly to combine. Continue to cook, covered, for about 5 minutes or until rice is tender and liquid is absorbed (add additional stock or water if needed).

5. Spoon rice-lobster mixture onto a heated serving platter or individual dishes. Garnish with cilantro or parsley and lemon slices and serve.

SERVES 4

Per serving: 275 calories; 15.5 grams protein; 45.5 grams carbohydrates; 3.7 grams fat; 41 milligrams cholesterol; 240 milligrams sodium (without salting).

GINGER AND LEMONGRASS-FLAVORED SCALLOPS ON RICE BED

Lemongrass is an herb and is one of the most important flavorings in Thai cooking. Because of its increased popularity, lemongrass is becoming more readily available in many large supermarkets, specialty greengrocers, and, of course, Asian markets. Look for long, thin, gray-green leaves and a scallion-like base. Lemongrass has a pleasantly sour-lemon flavor and fragrance, and lemon peel may be used as a substitute in a pinch.

This is one of the tastiest and most exotic dishes I've developed and it goes very well with a slightly sweet-sauced cucumber salad along with ice-cold beer or the traditional tea. Shrimps make a fine substitute for the scallops.

  1 stalk lemongrass, finely chopped
  2 tablespoons grated peeled ginger
  1 clove garlic, pressed
  1 tablespoon fresh lemon juice
  $^1/_2$ teaspoon hot pepper sauce or to taste
  $^1/_2$ pound sea scallops, each cut in half horizontally
  1 cup rice
  2 cups Low Fat Chicken Stock (page 3) or canned low sodium broth
    Salt and freshly ground pepper or to taste
  3 scallions, white and tender greens, thinly sliced
  2 plum tomatoes, seeded and diced

1. Combine lemongrass, ginger, garlic, lemon juice, and hot pepper sauce in a medium bowl and mix thoroughly. Add scallops to bowl and toss to combine. Refrigerate and let marinate for about 30 minutes, turning scallops once or twice.

2. While scallops marinate, combine rice, stock, and salt and pepper in a medium saucepan. Cover and cook over low heat for about 15 minutes or until rice is tender and liquid is absorbed; add additional stock or water if needed. Remove from heat and set aside.

3. Preheat broiler. Remove scallops from marinade and place in a broiler pan and broil for 2 to 3 minutes on each side, turning scallops once.

4. While scallops broil, add scallions to rice, toss lightly to just combine and heat for 1 minute. Remove rice from heat and fluff with fork.

5. Spoon rice onto a heated serving platter and top with broiled scallops. Garnish with tomatoes and serve immediately.

SERVES 4
Per serving: 240 calories; 13.5 grams protein; 42.0 grams carbohydrates; 1.7 grams fat; 22 milligrams cholesterol; 140 milligrams sodium (without salting).

MINTED BULGUR
WITH SPICY SHRIMP

Definitely not for the meek, this fabulous dish can bring tears to the eyes, fixing them in positions formerly unknown to human anatomy. So it's best to serve it only to fellow fire-eaters. Personally, I love hot food, so long as the underlying flavors are brightened, not overwhelmed.

$3/4$ pound medium shrimp, shelled, deveined, and
    rinsed
2 tablespoons hot pepper sauce or to taste
$1/2$ cup fine bulgur
4 cups water
1 small onion, minced
$1/4$ cup minced fresh mint leaves
2 teaspoons fresh lemon juice
2 tablespoons no-salt-added tomato juice
4 teaspoons olive oil
  Salt and freshly ground pepper to taste

1. Combine shrimp and hot sauce in a medium bowl and toss to combine. Cover and refrigerate until needed.

2. In a large bowl, combine bulgur and water. Allow bulgur to soak for 30 minutes. Drain and transfer to a colander that has been lined with a clean dishcloth. Draw cloth tightly together and squeeze out water. Transfer bulgur to a dry bowl.

3. Combine onion, mint, lemon juice, tomato

juice, and 2 teaspoons of the olive oil in a small bowl. Mix thoroughly and spoon gradually over bulgur. Season to taste with salt and pepper, then spoon onto a serving platter.

4. Heat remaining 2 teaspoons of oil in a medium nonstick skillet. Add shrimp and sauté over medium-high heat, turning shrimp to cook on all sides, for about 3 minutes or until cooked through. Using a slotted spoon, top bulgur with shrimp, and serve.

SERVES 4

Per serving: 210 calories; 20.0 grams protein; 18.0 grams carbohydrates; 6.5 grams fat; 130 milligrams cholesterol; 250 milligrams sodium (without salting).

THE MAIN DISH:
VEGETABLES

FUSILLI WITH DRIED TOMATOES, BASIL, AND RICOTTA

This dish is easy to make and always pleases. By using low fat cheeses the pasta tastes rich but is surprisingly low in fat.

¹/₂ cup unseasoned dried tomatoes (not oil-packed)
1 cup low fat ricotta cheese
2 tablespoons grated low fat Parmesan cheese (about 1 ounce)
*   Salt and freshly ground pepper to taste*
¹/₂ pound fusilli (corkscrew pasta)
¹/₂ cup slivered fresh basil leaves

1. Plump dried tomatoes in hot water. Drain and cut into slivers.

2. In a large serving bowl beat ricotta with Parmesan cheese until creamy. Stir in dried tomatoes and salt and pepper to taste and set aside.

3. Cook pasta in a large pot full of boiling water (salted, if desired) until al dente. Drain quickly and add to bowl with cheese-tomato mixture along with basil slivers. Toss to coat pasta.

4. Taste and correct seasonings if necessary and serve immediately.

SERVES 4

Per serving: 330 calories; 17.5 grams protein; 52.0 grams carbohydrates; 5.5 grams fat; 17 milligrams cholesterol; 140 milligrams sodium (without salting).

VEGETABLE PASTA
WITH ARTICHOKE HEARTS

Pastas come in a wide variety of colors and flavors, and are designed to please both the eye and palate of even the most jaded macaroni maven. Beet-flavored pasta is maroon; tomato, red bell pepper pasta and those flavored with fiery dried pepper flakes are, appropriately enough, red. Spinach, basil, and other herb pastas come in lovely shades of green, and carrots add sweetness and a wonderful golden hue to the pasta dough. Unusual nonvegetable-flavored pastas include lemon (yellow), which is terrific with spicy dishes and in salad, and there's a gorgeous black variety made with cuttlefish ink that's superb with shellfish-based sauces.

For the recipe described below, the more adventurous may wish to mix and match two or three different colors/flavors of pasta, or ready-packaged tricolored pasta will do very nicely.

1/2 pound vegetable pasta, any variety and shape
 2 teaspoons olive oil
 3 shallots, finely minced
1/4 cup dry vermouth
1/2 cup vegetable or chicken stock or broth
 1 package (9 ounces) frozen and thawed artichoke hearts, cut in half
1/4 teaspoon hot red pepper flakes or to taste

Salt to taste
3 tablespoons chopped fresh basil or parsley

1. Cook pasta in a large pot full of boiling water (salted, if desired) until al dente.

2. Heat oil in a large nonstick skillet. Add shallots and cook, stirring, for 1 minute. Add vermouth and stock, bring to a simmer and cook for an additional minute.

3. Add artichoke hearts to skillet. Stir, then remove from heat and set aside.

4. When pasta is cooked, drain and add to skillet. Season with red pepper flakes and salt to taste, toss to combine and heat through. Transfer ingredients to a platter, garnish with basil or parsley, and serve.

SERVES 4

Per serving: 265 calories; 9.0 grams protein; 49.0 grams carbohydrates; 3.5 grams fat; 0 milligrams cholesterol; 50 milligrams sodium (without salting).

SPICY EGGPLANT
AND ANGEL HAIR PASTA

The secret of this dish is to use either small Asian eggplant that are pale lavender, or the tiny deep purple Italian eggplant. These smaller eggplant are delicate in flavor rather than bitter, have fewer seeds, and do not need to be peeled.

4 small Asian or Italian eggplant (about 1 pound)
2 teaspoons olive oil
2 cloves garlic, pressed
1/4 teaspoon hot red pepper flakes or to taste
2 tablespoons balsamic vinegar
1 teaspoon sugar
Salt to taste
1/2 pound angel hair pasta
1 tablespoon grated low fat Parmesan cheese

1. Remove stems from eggplant and dice eggplant without peeling.

2. Heat oil in a large nonstick skillet. Add eggplant and sauté, stirring occasionally, for about 10 minutes or until eggplant has softened.

3. Add pepper flakes, vinegar, sugar, and salt to skillet. Stir to combine, then cover and simmer over low heat for about 10 minutes, or until eggplant is very soft.

4. While eggplant simmers, cook angel hair pasta in a large pot full of boiling water (salted, if desired) until al dente.

5. Drain pasta and transfer to a heated serving platter. Spoon eggplant mixture over pasta, sprinkle with Parmesan, and serve immediately.

SERVES 4

Per serving: 260 calories; 8.0 grams protein; 48.5 grams carbohydrates; 3.5 grams fat; 1 milligram cholesterol; 35 milligrams sodium (without salting).

TOMATO PASTA WITH ASPARAGUS

This recipe calls for any shaped pasta that's tomato-flavored—rotelle, fusilli, or small shells will work equally well. The contrast of the red pasta to the green vegetable makes the presentation something special.

1/2 pound tomato pasta, any shape
 1 pound asparagus, tough ends removed
 1 tablespoon fresh lemon juice
 2 teaspoons olive oil
 1 clove garlic, pressed
1/2 cup Low Fat Chicken Stock (page 3) or canned low
    .sodium broth
    Salt and freshly ground pepper to taste

1. Cook tomato pasta in a large pot full of boiling water (salted, if desired) until al dente.

2. While pasta cooks, place asparagus in one layer in a large skillet. Add water to cover and bring to a boil. Reduce heat to a simmer, cover, and cook until asparagus is just tender (depending on the age of the asparagus and your own preference this could be anywhere from 3 to 8 minutes). Remove asparagus from skillet and drain on paper towels. Discard water and dry skillet.

3. Heat oil in skillet. Add garlic and cook, stirring, for 1 minute. Add stock and salt and pepper. Stir to

combine, heat to a simmer, and cook for an additional minute. Remove from heat and set aside.

4. Cut drained asparagus diagonally into 1-inch lengths and season with lemon juice, and salt and pepper to taste and set aside.

5. When pasta is cooked, drain and add to skillet. Toss to combine and return to heat until ingredients are heated through.

6. Transfer pasta to a heated platter, top with asparagus, and serve immediately.

SERVES 4
Per serving: 245 calories; 9.0 grams protein; 44.0 grams carbohydrates; 3.7 grams fat; 1 milligram cholesterol; 20 milligrams sodium (without salting).

PAGLIA E FIENO

Paglia e Fieno means "straw and hay," and calls for two pastas—one white, the other green or spinach flavored. The combination is enhanced with peas and a dice of plum tomatoes for a colorful accent.

1/4 pound white fettuccine
1/4 pound green fettuccine
2 teaspoons olive oil
1/4 cup dry white wine
1/2 cup Low Fat Chicken Stock (page 3) or canned low sodium broth
1 cup fresh young green peas or frozen and thawed petite peas
Salt and freshly ground pepper to taste
2 plum tomatoes, diced

1. Cook pasta in a large pot full of boiling water (salted, if desired) until al dente.

2. While pasta cooks, heat oil in a large nonstick skillet. Add wine and bring to a boil. Reduce heat to medium-low and cook for 2 minutes.

3. Add stock and peas to skillet. Cover and cook for 4 to 5 minutes or until peas are just tender. Remove from heat and set aside.

4. When fettuccine is cooked, drain and transfer to a heated serving platter or large bowl. Spoon peas and sauce over fettuccine, season to taste with salt and pepper, and toss to combine. Garnish with tomatoes and serve.

SERVES 4

Per serving: 275 calories; 9.5 grams protein; 49.5 grams carbohydrates; 4.0 grams fat; 1 milligram cholesterol; 20 milligrams sodium (without salting).

PENNE WITH
GARLIC-AND-CHILI BROCCOLI

This straightforward dish really depends on the amount and strength of the chili powder you use. I think the more and the stronger the better, but it depends on how spicy you like your food.

  1 bunch broccoli, trimmed, cut into bite-size florets
 ½ pound penne
    Salt to taste
  1 tablespoon olive oil
  2 cloves garlic, pressed
  2 teaspoons chili powder or to taste
  2 tablespoons vegetable or chicken stock or broth

1. In a large saucepan, cover and steam broccoli florets in about 1 inch of water for about 10 minutes or until just tender. Drain and set aside.

2. Cook pasta in a large pot full of boiling water (salted, if desired) until al dente.

3. Heat oil in a large nonstick skillet. Add garlic and cook, stirring, for 2 minutes. Add broccoli to skillet and season with chili powder. Add stock and cook, stirring, for 2 minutes or until heated through.

4. When penne is cooked, add to skillet and toss with broccoli. Cover and heat through. Taste and correct seasoning, if necessary, before serving.

Serves 4
Per serving: 265 calories; 9.0 grams protein; 46.0 grams
carbohydrates; 5.0 grams fat; 0 milligrams cholesterol;
40 milligrams sodium (without salting).

EGG BARLEY
WITH WILD MUSHROOMS
AND SAGE

Egg barley is actually a small pasta that's barley-shaped. It may be purchased either toasted or untoasted, and while I find the toasted version more flavorful, the recipe can be prepared with either variety. If egg barley is unavailable, substitute pastini, orzo, or a similar small pasta.

This dish can be served immediately or refrigerated for a day or two, then warmed over very low heat before serving.

    1 tablespoon olive oil
 $^1/_2$ pound egg barley, preferably toasted
 $^1/_2$ pound wild mushrooms (oyster, portobello, morels,
        etc., or combination), wiped clean and thinly
        sliced
 $1^1/_2$ cups low sodium beef, chicken, or vegetable stock or
        broth
 $^1/_2$ teaspoon dried sage or to taste
    Salt and freshly ground pepper to taste
    2 tablespoons chopped fresh parsley

1. Heat oil in a heavy saucepan. Add egg barley and mushrooms and stir over medium-low heat for 2 minutes.

2. Add stock, sage, and salt and pepper to saucepan and stir to combine. Cover and cook over low heat for 15 to 20 minutes or until egg barley is

tender. Liquid should be completely absorbed by that time; if egg barley is not completely cooked, add additional stock or water.

3. Stir in parsley and correct seasoning if necessary. Transfer to a heated platter or bowl and serve immediately or refrigerate and reheat before serving.

SERVES 4

Per serving: 265 calories; 8.5 grams protein; 45.0 grams carbohydrates; 5.3 grams fat; 2 milligrams cholesterol; 34 milligrams sodium (without salting).

WILD RICE AND ZUCCHINI ROUNDS WITH WHITE BEANS

The idea for this dish came from a friend of mine from Georgia who uses the fresh and abundant zucchini in a variety of ways. In her hometown, where most of the zucchini is rolled in cornmeal and deep fried, this recipe is a breath of fresh—and greaseless—air.

Wild rice and zucchini is one of my favorite combinations, and the addition of the white beans makes it as toothsome as it is unconventional. It goes nicely with a delicate salad of baby lettuces drizzled with any herb-flavored vinegar.

1 1/2 cups low sodium vegetable or chicken stock or broth
1/4 cup dry white wine
1/2 cup water
3/4 cup wild rice, rinsed and drained
   Salt and freshly ground pepper to taste
1 tablespoon olive oil
3 small zucchini, ends trimmed and cut into thin
   rounds
1/2 teaspoon paprika or to taste
1/2 cup cooked or canned and drained small white
   beans
2 tablespoons chopped fresh Italian parsley

1. In a large saucepan, bring stock, wine, and water to a boil. Add rice and salt and pepper to taste. Stir to combine and return to a boil. Cover, reduce

heat to a simmer and cook for 30 to 45 minutes or until liquid is absorbed and rice is as tender as you prefer; add additional stock or water if needed.

2. While rice cooks, heat oil in a large nonstick skillet. Add zucchini, season with paprika, and cook over medium-high heat for about 5 minutes or until zucchini is lightly browned on both sides.

3. Add beans to skillet and stir to combine. Cook for 2 minutes or until heated through. Taste and adjust seasoning if necessary.

4. Spoon rice into a heated dish, top with zucchini rounds and beans, garnish with parsley, and serve.

SERVES 4
Per serving: 190 calories; 7.5 grams protein; 31.0 grams carbohydrates; 4.5 grams fat; 0 milligrams cholesterol; 30 milligrams sodium (without salting).

ASPARAGUS AND RICE
WITH ALMONDS

A green-and-golden combination that goes well with everything—but most beautifully with simply broiled salmon fillet and a salad of seasonal greens with a dash of fresh lemon or lime juice.

1 pound asparagus, tough stems removed
Salt and freshly ground pepper to taste
1 tablespoon olive oil
1 cup rice
1 1/2 cups low sodium vegetable or chicken stock or broth
1/2 cup water, approximate
1/2 teaspoon ground turmeric
1/2 teaspoon dried oregano
1 1/2 tablespoons blanched and slivered almonds
4 teaspoons chopped fresh chives

1. In a medium saucepan, cover asparagus in water and cook, covered, until crisp-tender. Drain, season to taste with salt and pepper, and set aside.

2. Heat oil in a large nonstick skillet or saucepan. Add rice and cook, stirring, for 1 minute. Add stock or broth to skillet, cover and cook over medium-low heat for 10 minutes.

3. Cut asparagus into 2-inch lengths. Add asparagus and almonds to rice and stir gently to combine. Add water, turmeric, and oregano and cook until rice is tender and liquid is absorbed (add additional

water if needed). Taste and correct seasoning. Sprinkle with chives and serve.

SERVES 4
Per serving: 245 calories; 6.5 grams protein; 41.0 grams carbohydrates; 6.1 grams fat; 0 milligrams cholesterol; 30 milligrams sodium (without salting).

SPINACH AND BASIL RISOTTO

To prepare an authentic Italian risotto it's best to use an Italian or short-grain rice. While this dish can be made with American long-grain rice, the stubby short grains absorb liquid more readily and the result is a dish with just the right texture.

4½ cups Low Fat Chicken Stock (page 3) or canned low
    sodium broth
1 tablespoon olive oil
6 shallots, minced
1 clove garlic, minced
1 cup arborio (Italian short-grain) rice
10 ounces spinach, washed, tough stems removed,
    chopped or shredded
¼ cup chopped fresh basil or 2 tablespoons dried
    Salt and freshly ground pepper to taste

1. Heat stock in a medium saucepan and keep at a slow simmer.

2. Heat oil in a large nonstick skillet or saucepan with a lid. Add shallots and garlic, and stir over medium heat for 1 minute or until slightly wilted. Add rice and salt and pepper and continue cooking and stirring for 2 minutes.

3. Pour a ladleful of simmering stock into rice mixture and cook, stirring, until liquid is absorbed.

4. Add the remainder of the stock to the rice gradually, a half cup at a time, waiting for the liquid to be absorbed before continuing. Stir in spinach, basil,

and salt and pepper to taste with the final half cup of liquid. Spinach and basil should be tender and rice should be creamy when all the stock is absorbed; add additional stock if needed.

5. Taste and adjust seasonings, if necessary, and serve immediately.

SERVES 4

Per serving: 255 calories; 6.5 grams protein; 45.0 grams carbohydrates; 5.5 grams fat; 23 milligrams cholesterol; 120 milligrams sodium (without salting).

POLENTA AND ZUCCHINI IN CREAMY DILL SAUCE

The neutral flavor of zucchini makes it an especially versatile vegetable. Here it is sautéed and seasoned with salt and wondrous paprika, which not only adds a delightful flavor but also gives the zucchini a lovely gold-rust hue. The tasty yogurt-dill sauce adds body making it the perfect topping for polenta. This dish would also be good using asparagus or green beans.

   2 teaspoons vegetable oil
   4 small zucchini, peeled and thinly sliced
   1/4 teaspoon hot paprika or to taste
      Salt to taste
   1 cup low fat plain yogurt
   1 teaspoon sugar
   2 tablespoons chopped fresh dill or 1 tablespoon dried
   4 cups water
   1 cup yellow cornmeal

1. Heat oil in a large nonstick skillet. Add zucchini, season with paprika and salt and cook, uncovered, stirring occasionally, for about 8 minutes or until zucchini is just tender.

2. Combine yogurt, sugar, and mix until well-blended. Spoon over zucchini and cook, stirring, for 2 minutes. Keep warm over low heat.

3. Heat water in a large saucepan, add salt if desired, and bring to a boil. Stir in cornmeal gradually

and cook, stirring frequently for 10 to 20 minutes or until polenta thickens.

4. Spoon polenta into a large, shallow bowl. Top with zucchini and sauce and serve immediately.

SERVES 4
Per serving: 175 calories; 6.5 grams protein; 28.5 grams carbohydrates; 4.3 grams fat; 4 milligrams cholesterol; 425 milligrams sodium (without salting).

VEGETABLE COUSCOUS
WITH CILANTRO

This dish with its Mideast flavor is a favorite with my vegetarian friends. And my nonvegetarian friends enjoy it when I serve it as a stuffing for chicken breasts.

    1 tablespoon olive oil
    2 cloves garlic, finely minced
    1 onion, finely diced
    1 stalk celery, diced
    1 carrot, finely diced
    1 small zucchini, finely diced
    4 large mushrooms, wiped clean and finely diced
 1½ cups low sodium vegetable stock or broth
    ½ teaspoon ground ginger
    ½ teaspoon ground coriander
    ¼ teaspoon ground cardamom
    ¼ teaspoon hot curry powder, optional
    1 cup quick-cooking couscous
    2 tablespoons chopped fresh cilantro
      Salt and freshly ground pepper to taste

1. Heat oil in a large nonstick skillet. Add garlic, onion, celery, carrot, zucchini, and mushrooms. Cook over medium heat, stirring frequently, for 5 minutes. Reduce heat to low, cover, and simmer for an additional 2 minutes.

2. Add stock, ginger, coriander, cardamom, and curry, if desired, to skillet. Stir to combine ingredi-

ents and bring to a boil. Reduce heat to medium, cover, and simmer for 5 minutes.

3. Stir couscous into skillet and bring to a rolling simmer. Cover and remove from heat. Let stand for 10 minutes.

4. Uncover and stir in cilantro and salt and pepper to taste, breaking up couscous with a fork. Serve immediately or let cool to room temperature.

SERVES 4
Per serving: 250 calories; 7.5 grams protein; 45.5 grams carbohydrates; 4.2 grams fat; 0 milligrams cholesterol; 50 milligrams sodium (without salting).

SIDE DISHES

PASTA WITH HERBED TOMATO SAUCE

Simple and delicious, this side dish goes well with almost anything—add some grated cheese and a small salad and it's a perfect main dish for two or three.

    1 teaspoon olive oil
    1 small onion, diced
    1 clove garlic, minced
    6 ripe plum tomatoes, chopped
    1 tablespoon no-salt-added tomato paste, preferably
        sun-dried
    1 tablespoon chopped fresh parsley or 1/2 tablespoon
        dried
    1/2 teaspoon each: dried thyme, marjoram, and oregano
        Salt and freshly ground pepper to taste
    6 ounces pasta of your choice

1. Heat oil in a medium saucepan. Add onion and garlic and stir over medium-low heat for 3 minutes.

2. Add all remaining ingredients, except pasta, to saucepan. Reduce heat to low and cook, stirring frequently, for 20 minutes.

3. When sauce is almost ready, cook pasta in a large pot full of boiling water (salted, if desired) until al dente.

4. Drain pasta and transfer to heated bowl. Add sauce and toss lightly to coat pasta. Serve immediately.

Per serving: 215 calories; 7.0 grams protein; 40.5 grams carbohydrates; 2.5 grams fat; 0 milligrams cholesterol; 25 milligrams sodium (without salting).

SMALL PASTA WITH UNCOOKED TOMATO SAUCE

Here's a great summer food when tomatoes are at their peak. I like to serve the pasta hot with this delicious sauce, but it can be made ahead and served at room temperature.

1½ pounds ripe fresh tomatoes, coarsely chopped, with juice
2 teaspoons fruity olive oil
2 tablespoons chopped fresh basil
1 clove garlic, smashed and minced
1 teaspoon minced hot green chili, optional
  Salt and freshly ground pepper to taste
½ pound tubettini or other small pasta, such as elbows or ditalini

1. Combine all ingredients, except pasta, in a large serving bowl. Stir or toss to blend and let stand at room temperature while pasta cooks.

2. Cook pasta in a medium saucepan full of boiling water (salted, if desired) until al dente.

3. Drain pasta and transfer to tomato mixture in bowl. Toss and serve.

SERVES 6
Per serving: 175 calories; 5.5 grams protein; 32.5 grams carbohydrates; 2.5 grams fat; 0 milligrams cholesterol; 20 milligrams sodium (without salting).

LINGUINE WITH GARLIC AND FRESH PARSLEY

I think this longtime favorite is just as delicious without the traditional half cup of oil. I also find adding a little wine vinegar imparts a flavorful tartness.

    1 tablespoon olive oil
    1 small onion, finely minced
    3 cloves garlic, finely minced
      Salt and freshly ground pepper to taste
    1/2 pound linguine
    3/4 cup Low Fat Chicken Stock (page 3) or canned low
        sodium broth
    1 tablespoon red wine vinegar
    1/2 cup packed chopped fresh Italian parsley leaves
    1 tablespoon chopped fresh Italian parsley

1. Heat oil in a large skillet. Add onion and garlic and cook over medium heat, stirring frequently, for 3 minutes or until onion is wilted. Do not let garlic brown. Season to taste with salt and pepper.

2. Meanwhile, cook linguine in a large pot full of boiling water (salt, if desired) until al dente.

3. Add stock and vinegar to skillet with onion and garlic and bring to a boil. Reduce heat to medium-high and simmer, uncovered, for 5 minutes or until stock is reduced slightly. Add 1/2 cup parsley and simmer for an additional 2 minutes.

4. Drain pasta and transfer to a heated serving

bowl. Add contents of skillet and toss lightly to coat pasta. Sprinkle with remaining tablespoon of parsley and serve.

SERVES 6

Per serving: 170 calories; 5.0 grams protein; 29.5 grams carbohydrates; 3.2 grams fat; 1 milligram cholesterol; 20 milligrams sodium (without salting).

FETTUCCINE WITH CREAMY CILANTRO PESTO

A kicky side dish with a fragrant and appealing
"pesto" sauce for pasta. "Pesto" is in quotes because, of course, fresh basil, oodles of olive oil and
Parmesan, and toasted pine nuts comprise the
traditional Genovese pesto. But my version is low
fat—and knockout sensational, too! For those who
have an aversion to cilantro, substitute a combination of fresh basil and parsley.

    6 ounces fettuccine or linguine
    ¾ cup low fat (1%) cottage cheese
    ½ cup packed fresh cilantro leaves
       Salt to taste
    1 tablespoon olive oil
    4 cloves garlic, thinly sliced
    ¼ teaspoon hot red pepper flakes or to taste

1. Cook pasta in a large pot full of boiling water
(salted, if desired) until al dente. Drain and set aside.
2. While pasta cooks, place cottage cheese, cilantro, and salt in a blender or food processor and process until smooth. Set aside.
3. Heat oil in a large nonstick skillet. Add garlic
and pepper flakes and cook over very low heat for
about 5 minutes or until garlic is golden. Remove
skillet from heat.
4. Add pasta and cheese mixture to skillet with

garlic. Toss until all ingredients are combined and serve immediately.

SERVES 4
Per serving: 225 calories; 11.0 grams protein; 33.5 grams carbohydrates; 4.8 grams fat; 2 milligrams cholesterol; 180 milligrams sodium (without salting).

CELLOPHANE NOODLES AND MIXED MUSHROOMS

This is my take on a Lohan (Buddhist) vegetarian dish with its basis in mushrooms. Here, I've used three types of mushrooms with just a few vegetables for color, but go ahead and use more if you wish. Any combination of wild and/or cultivated mushrooms will work well.

6 ounces cellophane noodles or angel hair pasta
2 teaspoons vegetable or olive oil
2 cloves garlic, thinly sliced
1 carrot, thinly sliced or shredded
10 snow peas, trimmed and stringed
6 dried shiitake mushrooms, soaked in hot water for
    20 minutes and cut in half
10 small button mushrooms, wiped clean
1 large portobello mushroom cap or 6 straw
    mushrooms, wiped clean and sliced
1 tablespoon Asian fish sauce (nam pla) or low
    sodium soy sauce
1 tablespoon cornstarch
1³/₄ cups water
1¹/₂ teaspoons sugar or to taste
1 teaspoon dry sherry
¹/₂ tablespoon rice wine vinegar

1. Cook noodles in a large pot full of boiling water (salted, if desired) until al dente. Drain.
2. While noodles cook, heat oil in a large nonstick

skillet or wok. Add garlic and cook over medium heat until golden. Add carrot and snow peas and cook, stirring, for 1 or 2 minutes to combine flavors. Add mushrooms and stir for another 2 minutes.

3. Dissolve cornstarch in water and add to skillet. Stir in fish sauce and simmer, stirring, for 2 minutes. Add sugar, sherry, and vinegar and stir for an additional 2 minutes or until thickened.

4. Transfer noodles to a serving platter or bowl. Spoon mushrooms and sauce from skillet over noodles and serve.

SERVES 4

Per serving: 225 calories; 2.0 grams protein; 48.5 grams carbohydrates; 2.5 grams fat; 0 milligrams cholesterol; 165 milligrams sodium (without salting).

SAFFRON RICE

The pimientos add their brilliant color and delectable flavor to this festive side dish. I also like small green peas (about a quarter cup should suffice) with this saffron-scented, very ritzy rice. It is extraordinary with grilled fish or a roasted chicken.

  2 teaspoons vegetable oil
  4 scallions, white and tender greens, thinly sliced
  1 stalk celery, thinly sliced
  1 clove garlic, finely minced, optional
  1/4 teaspoon crumbled saffron threads or to taste
  1 cup rice
  2 cups Low Fat Chicken Stock (page 3), vegetable
      broth, or water
    Salt and freshly ground pepper to taste
1 1/2 tablespoons minced pimientos

1. Heat oil in a large nonstick pot. Add scallions, celery, and garlic if desired. Stir over medium heat for 3 to 4 minutes or until vegetables are slightly wilted.

2. Add saffron and rice to pot and stir briefly to coat rice. Add stock and season to taste with salt and pepper. Bring to a boil, cover, reduce heat to low, and simmer gently for about 20 minutes or until rice is tender.

3. Transfer rice to a heated serving bowl or platter, add pimientos, and fluff with fork before serving.

Per serving: 140 calories; 3.0 grams protein; 26.0 grams carbohydrates; 2.3 grams fat; 2 milligrams cholesterol; 30 milligrams sodium (without salting).

RISOTTO WITH BLACK OLIVES

This recipe uses the traditional way of preparing risotto, except, of course, my rendition calls for just the bare minimum of oil. Labor-intensive? You bet. But you'll wind up with a dish that is delectably creamy while the grains remain separate and firm. The addition of black (ripe) olives leaves distinctive marks of color, texture, and rich taste.

A salad of Belgian endive, watercress or arugula and radicchio would be enough for a most memorable light lunch.

3¹/₂ cups Low Fat Chicken Stock (page 3) or canned low
    sodium broth, approximate
 ¹/₂ cup dry white wine
  1 tablespoon olive oil
  1 onion, finely minced
 ³/₄ cup arborio (Italian short-grain) rice
    Salt and freshly ground pepper to taste
  1 ounce pitted black olives, preferably gaeta or
    calamata, coarsely chopped
    Grated low fat Parmesan cheese to taste, optional

1. Combine stock and wine in a medium saucepan and bring to a boil. Reduce heat to low and keep at a slow simmer.

2. Heat oil in a large, heavy nonstick saucepan or deep skillet. Add onion and stir over medium heat for 2 minutes or until slightly wilted. Add rice and

salt and pepper to taste. Stir for 1 to 2 minutes or until rice is coated and just starts to turn golden.

3. Pour in a ladleful of simmering stock into rice mixture and cook, stirring, until liquid is absorbed. Promptly add another ladleful of stock and repeat procedure. Continue until stock is nearly used up and rice is creamy.

4. Stir olives into rice and continue to stir, adding any leftover stock, until rice is very creamy. Taste and adjust seasonings, if necessary. Serve hot with grated cheese on the side if desired.

SERVES 4

Per serving: 205 calories; 4.0 grams protein; 34.5 grams carbohydrates; 5.7 grams fat; 5 milligrams cholesterol; 125 milligrams sodium (without salting).

SOUTHWESTERN GRITS

Here's a hot idea for an unusual, low fat side dish, midday snack, or breakfast dish using quick-cooking grits, vegetables, and jalapeño chilies.

I prefer creamy grits so my recipe calls for two cups of stock; for a firmer texture, use 1¾ cups stock or to taste.

½ tablespoon vegetable oil
2 scallions, white and 2-inch greens, thinly sliced
2 tablespoons diced red bell pepper, with seeds
1 teaspoon minced jalapeño pepper or to taste
1½ ounces very lean Canadian bacon or smoked lean ham, diced
Salt and freshly ground pepper to taste
2 cups Low Fat Chicken Stock (page 3) or canned low sodium broth
½ cup quick-cooking grits
¼ cup water

1. Heat oil in small nonstick skillet. Add scallions, bell pepper, and jalapeño pepper and sauté over medium heat, stirring, for 2 to 3 minutes or until peppers soften.

2. Add bacon or ham to skillet, reduce heat to low and cook for an additional 2 minutes. Season to taste with salt and pepper and set aside.

3. Heat stock in a large nonstick saucepan and bring to a boil. Add grits and cook for 10 minutes, stirring frequently.

4. Add contents of skillet to saucepan with grits. Mix thoroughly to combine ingredients and cook over low heat for 2 minutes.

5. Meanwhile, deglaze skillet with $1/4$ cup water and add to grits mixture. Stir well and serve immediately.

SERVES 4

Per serving: 115 calories; 4.5 grams protein; 17.0 grams carbohydrates; 3.5 grams fat; 8 milligrams cholesterol; 200 milligrams sodium (without salting).

CORN BREAD

Corn bread complements grilled meats and poultry and fish. It also goes extremely well with all Mexican and Southwestern foods—and, of course, it's a standard side dish at Southern meals.

This simple-but-deliciously versatile corn bread can be further enhanced by adding a tablespoon or two of shredded cheddar cheese and/or finely minced jalapeños to the batter.

1 cup yellow cornmeal
1/2 cup all-purpose flour
1 1/2 teaspoons double-acting baking powder
1/4 teaspoon baking soda
1/4 teaspoon salt
   Egg substitute equal to 2 eggs
1 cup low fat buttermilk
1/2 stick unsalted butter or margarine, melted and cool

1. Preheat oven to 350° F.

2. Combine cornmeal, flour, baking powder, baking soda, and salt in a medium bowl and whisk together.

3. In a separate bowl, combine egg substitute, buttermilk, and butter or margarine and whisk together. Add egg mixture to cornmeal mixture, mixing until the batter is just combined. Do not overblend.

4. Spoon batter into a nonstick 8-inch baking pan. Bake for 25 to 30 minutes or until corn bread is

springy to the touch and pulls away from the side of the pan.

  5. Allow to cool before cutting into squares.

MAKES 16 SQUARES
Per square: 65 calories; 2.0 grams protein; 9.0 grams carbohydrates; 2.5 grams fat; 6 milligrams cholesterol; 200 milligrams sodium.

DESSERTS

PASTA AND RICE DESSERTS

Noodle desserts are popular and well-loved in eastern Europe, while rice pudding is an all-American favorite. The desserts presented here are simple to prepare, and make a wonderful finale to a light meal or a salad lunch.

LASAGNA BAKED WITH
FRESH PLUMS

Cardamom is a member of the ginger family with a pungent aroma and a warm, spicy-sweet flavor. This spice is widely used in Scandinavian and East Indian cooking with a light and knowing hand because a little goes a long way.

Try this fragrant dessert very warm, with a dollop of cold vanilla yogurt or fat-free ice cream.

1½ cups pitted and sliced ripe fresh plums
1 tablespoon sugar
¼ cup orange juice
⅛ teaspoon ground cardamom
½ pound lasagna noodles
    Vegetable oil cooking spray

1. Combine plums, sugar, juice, and cardamom in a medium heavy saucepan. Cook, uncovered, until plums have thickened into a sauce. Remove from heat and reserve.

2. Preheat oven to 350° F.

3. Cook pasta in a large pot full of boiling water (salted, if desired) until al dente. Drain and let cool. Cut each noodle in half.

4. Using a nonstick baking pan lightly coated with cooking spray, create layers of noodles and plums, starting and finishing with plums. Cover dish with foil and bake for 10 to 15 minutes or until ingredients are heated through.

5. Remove from oven and let cool slightly. Cut into squares before serving.

<small>SERVES</small> 6
Per serving: 185 calories; 5.5 grams protein; 37.0 grams carbohydrates; 1.5 grams fat; 0 milligrams cholesterol; 10 milligrams sodium.

FARFALLE WITH PEARS AND WALNUTS

I often call this "Bartlett and bows," because I usually use this succulent variety of pear for cooking. If you can't find the perfect pair of pears, substitute apples.

1/2 pound farfalle (small pasta bows)
1 tablespoon fresh lemon juice
2 small just-ripe pears, peeled, cored, and coarsely grated
2 tablespoons ground walnuts
1 tablespoon sugar

1. Cook pasta in a large pot full of boiling water (salted, if desired) until al dente. Drain and transfer to a serving bowl.

2. Sprinkle lemon juice over grated pears in a small bowl. Toss to combine and set aside.

3. Combine walnuts and sugar in a small bowl and mix well.

4. Add walnut-sugar combination to pasta and toss. Transfer to dessert plates, top each with an equal amount of shredded pears, and serve.

SERVES 4
Per serving: 265 calories; 8.0 grams protein; 51.0 grams carbohydrates; 3.2 grams fat; 0 milligrams cholesterol; 10 milligrams sodium.

BROAD NOODLES
TOSSED WITH COTTAGE CHEESE

This is an abbreviated (but no less delicious) version of "luchen kugel," or noodle pudding, using about a cup less butter. If you like, strew a few plumped-in-wine raisins on top or dust yogurt with cinnamon-sugar.

1/2 cup low fat cottage cheese
2 teaspoons sugar
1 teaspoon grated lemon rind
1/2 pound broad noodles
2 teaspoons unsalted butter or margarine
1/2 cup low fat vanilla yogurt

1. Combine cottage cheese, sugar, and lemon rind in a small bowl. Mix well and set aside (do not refrigerate).

2. Cook pasta in a large pot full of boiling water (salted, if desired) until al dente.

3. When noodles are almost cooked, heat butter or margarine in a large nonstick skillet.

4. Drain noodles and transfer to skillet with butter. Toss to coat noodles and remove from heat.

5. Spoon cottage cheese mixture over noodles and toss again.

6. Transfer noodles to dessert plates. Garnish with a dollop of yogurt and serve.

SERVES 4

Per serving: 285 calories; 13.0 grams protein; 47.0 grams carbohydrates; 5.0 grams fat; 57 milligrams cholesterol; 165 milligrams sodium.

ORECCHIETTE WITH APRICOT AND APPLE

Orecchiette are tiny discs of pasta that have an ear-like shape. Try this quick and easy dessert—it looks as luscious as it tastes.

¼ cup low sugar apricot fruit spread
½ cup apple juice
½ pound orecchiette pasta

1. Combine apricot fruit spread and apple juice in a small, heavy saucepan. Warm over low heat, stirring to combine. Remove from heat and keep warm by placing saucepan on a range-proof trivet.

2. Cook orecchiette in a medium pot full of boiling water (salted, if desired) until al dente. Drain and place in a serving bowl.

3. Spoon apricot-apple mixture over pasta, toss to combine, and serve immediately.

SERVES 4
Per serving: 245 calories; 7.0 grams protein; 51.0 grams carbohydrates; 1.0 grams fat; 0 milligrams cholesterol; 10 milligrams sodium.

ORANGE-FLAVORED
RICE DESSERT

Here's a variation on an old theme—rice pudding that is rich in flavor without depending on cream or whole eggs.

  1 cup evaporated skim milk
  1 cup rice
  2 cups low fat (1%) milk
  1 tablespoon sugar
  1 teaspoon grated orange rind
  1/4 cup orange juice

1. Pour evaporated milk into a small bowl and place in freezer for at least 1 hour or until slush forms on edges. Freeze beaters as well.

2. Combine rice, milk, and sugar in a medium heavy saucepan and bring to a boil. Cover, reduce and simmer until liquid is absorbed and rice is tender. Remove from heat and set aside to cool.

3. While rice cooks, beat evaporated milk until stiff.

4. Stir orange rind and orange juice into cooked rice, then fold in the beaten evaporated milk.

5. Spoon mixture into a dessert bowl or soufflé dish. Refrigerate overnight or for about 8 hours before serving.

SERVES 4

Per serving: 295 calories; 12.5 grams protein; 56.5 grams
carbohydrates; 1.8 grams fat; 8 milligrams cholesterol;
140 milligrams sodium.

COLD RICE PUDDING
TOPPED WITH FRESH BERRIES

For a nice alternative, use fresh seedless oranges, mandarin oranges, or petite clementines, combining them with Grand Marnier or another orange-flavored liqueur, or juice.

1 cup rice
2¼ cups low fat (2%) milk
2 tablespoons sugar
1 envelope unflavored gelatin
¼ cup water
2 tablespoons low fat sour cream
1 cup fresh berries (raspberries, blackberries, strawberries, or combination), coarsely chopped
1 tablespoon port or Madeira wine, optional

1. Combine rice, milk, and sugar in a medium heavy saucepan and bring to a boil. Cover and reduce heat to very low. Simmer until liquid is absorbed; rice should be tender and creamy.

2. Soften the gelatin in water and heat in a double boiler until liquid is clear. Add gelatin to rice mixture and stir until ingredients are combined. Set aside to cool until pudding is just thickened.

3. Fold sour cream into the rice mixture and spoon into dessert dishes. Chill until firm.

4. Just before serving, combine berries with port or Madeira, if desired, in a small saucepan and heat to a simmer. Remove from heat and let cool.

5. Garnish each portion with berry topping and serve.

SERVES 6
Per serving: 195 calories; 6.5 grams protein; 36.0 grams carbohydrates; 2.5 grams fat; 9 milligrams cholesterol; 55 milligrams sodium.

RASPBERRY-RICE PARFAIT WITH CANDIED GINGER

Rich, but not overly sweet, serve this gorgeous-colored dessert in stemmed glasses for a festive finale to any meal.

    1 cup rice
    2 cups low fat (1%) milk
    2 teaspoons sugar
    ½ teaspoon vanilla extract
    ½ cup frozen raspberries in syrup, thawed
    ½ ounce crystallized ginger, minced

1. In a medium heavy saucepan combine rice, milk, sugar, and vanilla extract and bring to a boil. Stir and reduce heat to low. Cover and simmer for 15 to 20 minutes or until rice is tender and liquid has been absorbed. Remove from heat and set aside to cool.

2. Prepare this dessert by layering raspberries and rice in parfait or champagne glasses. The first layer should be raspberries and the last rice.

3. Garnish the top of each dessert with crystallized ginger and serve at room temperature or chilled.

SERVES 4
Per serving: 280 calories; 7.5 grams protein; 56.0 grams carbohydrates; 2.5 grams fat; 9 milligrams cholesterol; 65 milligrams sodium.

BAKED RICE CAKE
WITH STRAWBERRY SAUCE

This rice cake bears no resemblance to the packaged rounds—but it is a great-tasting low fat treat.

1 cup rice
4 1/2 cups low fat (1%) milk
3 1/2 tablespoons sugar
    Egg substitute equal to 2 eggs
1/2 teaspoon vanilla extract
2 egg whites, stiffly beaten
1/2 cup fresh strawberries
2 tablespoons crushed ice

1. In a large heavy saucepan combine rice and 4 cups milk. Bring to a boil. Reduce heat to a simmer and add 2 tablespoons of sugar. Stir to combine, cover, and cook for 15 minutes. Remove rice from heat and set aside to cool.

2. Preheat oven to 325° F.

3. Combine egg substitute with 1 tablespoon sugar. Add vanilla extract and beat until blended.

4. Stir egg mixture into rice-milk combination and fold in beaten egg whites.

5. Spoon rice mixture into a 12-inch-square nonstick cake pan and bake for about 45 minutes or until set. Remove from oven and let cool slightly.

6. Before serving, combine remaining 1/2 cup milk, 1/2 tablespoon sugar, strawberries, and crushed ice in

a blender. Blend at high speed until ice is crushed and ingredients have thickened.

7. Cut rice cake into 6 squares and serve with sauce.

SERVES 6

Per serving: 235 calories; 11.5 grams protein; 42.0 grams carbohydrates; 2.2 grams fat; 8 milligrams cholesterol; 140 milligrams sodium.

INDEX